GREEN LIVING FOR A HEALTHY MIND AND BODY: SUSTAINABLE PRACTICES FOR WELLNESS

INTRODUCTION

Welcome to Green Life, Healthy Life—a guide to transforming your well-being while creating a positive impact on the planet. In these pages, you'll discover that living sustainably isn't just about recycling or buying eco-friendly products; it's a deeply enriching approach to life that fosters personal health, mental clarity, and a lasting sense of purpose. Here, we'll explore the powerful connection between a green lifestyle and a vibrant, balanced life that benefits both you and the world around you.
As we face climate challenges, pollution, and a fast-paced society, sustainable living offers more than just a chance to "help the Earth." It presents us with a unique path to improve our lives, reconnect with nature, and find peace in simplicity. Imagine starting each day with a renewed sense of energy, knowing that each choice—from the food you eat to the products you use—reflects a commitment to both your health and the well-being of the planet. By incorporating eco-friendly habits, you'll discover a profound shift in how you feel physically, emotionally, and mentally.

In *Green Life, Healthy Life*, we'll explore a range of sustainable practices that can enhance your life in meaningful ways:

- **Eating for Health and Sustainability**: We'll dive into the world of eco-friendly diets, focusing on the power of fresh, whole foods that not only fuel your body but also reduce your environmental footprint. You'll learn how to choose ingredients that nourish you and respect the Earth, helping you feel energized and balanced.

- **Reducing Environmental Toxins**: Many products we encounter daily, from cleaning supplies to personal care items, contain chemicals that may be harmful to our health. Here, we'll uncover ways to minimize these environmental stressors, enabling you to create a home that feels cleaner and healthier. Imagine breathing easier, feeling less drained, and enjoying a more vibrant living space—all by making small, sustainable adjustments.

- **Nature's Healing Power**: Did you know that simply spending time outside can improve your mental well-being? Nature has a way of calming our minds, reducing stress, and even enhancing creativity. We'll look at practical ways to connect with nature, whether it's through a daily walk, setting up a green space at home, or exploring the natural world around you. Even brief encounters with nature can create a sense of peace and clarity that's difficult to find in today's busy world.

- **Sustainable Living and Mental Health**: As our lives become increasingly connected to screens, noise, and endless tasks, many of us crave simplicity and mindfulness. Sustainable living encourages a return to meaningful moments and intentional choices, both of which are beneficial for mental health. By adopting a lifestyle that's in harmony with the Earth, you'll discover an inner calm and resilience, reducing stress and anxiety while boosting a sense of accomplishment and purpose.

This book isn't about extreme changes or sacrificing comfort for a noble cause. It's about discovering a way of life that brings you closer to your best self while respecting the planet. Each chapter provides simple, actionable steps that you can take immediately, building a foundation for a healthier life and a healthier planet. You'll find stories of those who've embraced green living, tips for incorporating eco-friendly habits into your busy schedule, and guidance on sustaining these changes in the long run.

Whether you're new to sustainability or already passionate about eco-friendly practices, *Green Life, Healthy Life* is a journey into a lifestyle that can elevate your physical health, mental clarity, and sense of fulfillment. Through this path, you'll gain more than knowledge—you'll gain a refreshed perspective on living fully and responsibly.

So, if you're ready to nurture both yourself and the planet, join me as we explore the countless ways that sustainable choices can bring balance, vitality, and joy into your everyday life. Let's embark on this exciting journey together, discovering that a green life is truly a path to a healthier, happier life.

Chapter 2: Nourishing Your Body, Nourishing the Planet

In a world where fast food is readily available and processed foods dominate store shelves, it can be easy to overlook the profound impact that our dietary choices have on both our health and the planet. Eating in a way that respects the Earth can nurture not only our bodies but also our environment. By making conscious choices in our diets, we can boost our energy levels, reduce the risk of chronic illness, and cultivate a more balanced lifestyle—all while helping to protect the planet for future generations.

In this chapter, we'll explore how to make food choices that are both healthy for us and sustainable for the Earth. You'll learn about the benefits of plant-forward diets, the importance of buying local and seasonal foods, and practical ways to minimize food waste. Together, these changes can create a more mindful, health-centered approach to eating that aligns with our natural environment.

Understanding the Impact of Our Food Choices

To understand sustainable eating, it's helpful to think of our food system as a cycle that connects many parts of life: from the soil where food is grown to the people who harvest it, from transportation to packaging, and from our plates to waste disposal. Each step of this cycle influences our health and the environment. When we consume heavily processed foods, eat large amounts of meat, or frequently throw away leftovers, we contribute to greenhouse gas emissions, habitat destruction, and pollution—all factors that degrade our health over time.

However, by opting for foods that are responsibly sourced, minimally processed, and closer to nature, we can help reduce these harmful effects. And as we'll see, sustainable eating doesn't have to be complicated. It's about making small, thoughtful choices that align with both our physical well-being and the health of the planet.

The Benefits of a Plant-Forward Diet

One of the most powerful changes we can make is to adopt a plant-forward diet. This doesn't mean you have to become fully vegetarian or vegan, but rather that plant-based foods make up the majority of your meals. Fruits, vegetables, grains, legumes, nuts, and seeds are naturally rich in nutrients like fiber, vitamins, and antioxidants, which support immune health, digestion, and energy levels.

Why Plant-Forward Eating Supports Health

- **High in Nutrients**: Plant-based foods are loaded with vitamins, minerals, and antioxidants that promote cellular health, strengthen the immune system, and reduce inflammation.

- **Supports Heart Health**: Diets rich in fruits, vegetables, whole grains, and legumes have been shown to lower blood pressure and cholesterol, reducing the risk of heart disease.

- **Improves Digestion**: The fiber in plants aids digestion, supports gut health, and promotes a feeling of fullness, which can help prevent overeating.

- **Weight Management**: Plant-based foods are often lower in calories yet filling, helping with healthy weight management.

Environmental Benefits of a Plant-Forward Diet

Beyond personal health, plant-based eating has a significant positive impact on the planet:

- **Lower Greenhouse Gas Emissions**: Plant-based foods have a lower carbon footprint compared to animal products, as they require less energy, water, and land to produce.

- **Reduces Deforestation**: Much of the world's deforestation is driven by the need for more land for livestock. By eating more plants, we help reduce the demand for new grazing land, thus preserving forests.

- **Less Water Usage**: Growing plants generally requires far less water than raising animals, which supports water conservation efforts.

Simple Ways to Start Eating More Plant-Based

1. **Choose One Plant-Based Meal a Day**: Try swapping one meal each day for a plant-based option. Start with something simple, like oatmeal with fruit for breakfast or a salad loaded with vegetables and legumes for lunch.

2. **Experiment with Meat Alternatives**: Enjoy new recipes with lentils, chickpeas, tofu, or tempeh as a protein source.

3. **Add More Vegetables to Your Plate**: Increase the portion of vegetables in each meal. You don't have to remove other foods entirely; just focus on adding more plants.

Embracing Local and Seasonal Eating

Eating locally and seasonally isn't just a fun way to explore new flavors; it's also one of the most effective ways to reduce the environmental impact of our diet.

Benefits of Local Eating

- **Reduces Carbon Emissions**: Local foods travel shorter distances, which means less fuel is used for transportation.

- **Supports the Local Economy**: Buying from local farmers helps strengthen the community and provides direct support to local businesses.

- **Fresher Produce**: Local fruits and vegetables are often fresher and tastier since they're harvested closer to their peak ripeness.

Why Seasonal Eating Matters

Seasonal eating means choosing foods that are naturally ready to harvest in your area at certain times of the year. It supports environmental sustainability because:

- **It Requires Less Energy**: Seasonal produce grows in harmony with natural conditions, requiring less artificial energy, like heating for greenhouses.

- **Reduces Food Waste**: Seasonal foods are usually more abundant, affordable, and less likely to spoil before reaching consumers, leading to less food waste.

Ways to Start Eating Locally and Seasonally

1. **Visit Farmers' Markets**: Local farmers' markets are a great

place to find fresh, seasonal produce, often grown without excessive pesticides.

2. **Research Seasonal Produce**: Make a list of fruits and vegetables available in your region each season. Use it as a guide for meal planning.

3. **Join a Community Supported Agriculture (CSA) Program**: CSA programs allow you to receive regular deliveries of seasonal produce from local farms, often with variety and freshness unmatched by grocery stores.

Mindful Consumption: Reducing Food Waste

Approximately one-third of all food produced globally is wasted, which contributes to greenhouse gas emissions and squanders resources like water and energy. By making a few small adjustments, we can significantly reduce food waste.

Steps to Reduce Food Waste

- **Plan Meals**: Plan your meals for the week, which helps avoid impulse purchases and food that ends up unused.

- **Store Food Properly**: Many fruits and vegetables last longer if stored correctly. For example, refrigerating apples and carrots keeps them fresh for weeks.

- **Use "Scraps" Wisely**: Many vegetable scraps can be saved for soups, sauces, or even homemade vegetable broth.

- **Embrace Leftovers**: Leftovers can be a convenient, waste-free meal option. Try incorporating them into a new dish, like turning roast vegetables into a salad or pasta.

The Personal and Environmental Benefits of Reducing Food Waste

- **Reduces Greenhouse Gas Emissions**: When food waste decomposes in landfills, it releases methane, a potent greenhouse gas. By reducing waste, we help mitigate climate change.

- **Saves Money**: By buying only what you need and making use of leftovers, you can save significantly on grocery bills.

- **Fosters a Gratitude for Food**: Being mindful of waste fosters a deeper appreciation for food, from the farmers who grow it to the journey it takes to reach your plate.

Putting It All Together: Crafting a Sustainable Diet That Works for You

Creating a sustainable, health-supporting diet doesn't mean overhauling everything overnight. It's about gradually incorporating new habits and being intentional with each choice. Here's a step-by-step guide to get started:

1. **Set Small Goals**: Begin with one or two changes, like adding a plant-based meal or shopping at a farmers' market once a week.

2. **Experiment with Recipes**: Find joy in the process by trying new recipes and cooking techniques. Sustainable eating should be enjoyable, not restrictive.

3. **Reflect on Your Journey**: Track how you feel as you make these changes. Many people find that eco-friendly eating improves their energy, digestion, and overall mood.

4. **Stay Open to Growth**: Remember, sustainable eating is a journey, not a fixed destination. Continue to learn about new practices, experiment with seasonal foods, and evolve your diet over time.

Conclusion

Eating in a way that nourishes both your body and the planet can transform not only your health but also your relationship with food. Each choice—from selecting more plants to reducing food waste—has a positive impact that goes far beyond the dining table. As you continue on this journey, remember that sustainable eating is not about being perfect. It's about making choices that align with your values, benefit your well-being, and support the Earth.

With each mindful bite, you're contributing to a healthier you and a healthier planet.

CHAPTER 2: NOURISHING YOUR BODY, NOURISHING THE PLANET

In a world where fast food is readily available and processed foods dominate store shelves, it can be easy to overlook the profound impact that our dietary choices have on both our health and the planet. Eating in a way that respects the Earth can nurture not only our bodies but also our environment. By making conscious choices in our diets, we can boost our energy levels, reduce the risk of chronic illness, and cultivate a more balanced lifestyle—all while helping to protect the planet for future generations.

In this chapter, we'll explore how to make food choices that are both healthy for us and sustainable for the Earth. You'll learn about the benefits of plant-forward diets, the importance of buying local and seasonal foods, and practical ways to minimize food waste. Together, these changes can create a more mindful, health-centered approach to eating that aligns with our natural environment.

Understanding the Impact of Our Food Choices

To understand sustainable eating, it's helpful to think of our food system as a cycle that connects many parts of life: from the soil where food is grown to the people who harvest it, from transportation to packaging, and from our plates to waste disposal. Each step of this cycle influences our health and the environment. When we consume heavily processed foods, eat large amounts of meat, or frequently throw away leftovers, we contribute to greenhouse gas emissions, habitat destruction, and pollution—all factors that degrade our health over time.

However, by opting for foods that are responsibly sourced, minimally processed, and closer to nature, we can help reduce these harmful effects. And as we'll see, sustainable eating doesn't have to be complicated. It's about making small, thoughtful choices that align with both our physical well-being and the health of the planet.

The Benefits of a Plant-Forward Diet

One of the most powerful changes we can make is to adopt a plant-forward diet. This doesn't mean you have to become fully vegetarian or vegan, but rather that plant-based foods make up the majority of your meals. Fruits, vegetables, grains, legumes, nuts, and seeds are naturally rich in nutrients like fiber, vitamins, and antioxidants, which support immune health, digestion, and energy levels.

Why Plant-Forward Eating Supports Health

- **High in Nutrients**: Plant-based foods are loaded with vitamins, minerals, and antioxidants that promote cellular health, strengthen the immune system, and reduce inflammation.

- **Supports Heart Health**: Diets rich in fruits, vegetables, whole grains, and legumes have been shown to lower blood pressure and cholesterol, reducing the risk of heart disease.

- **Improves Digestion**: The fiber in plants aids digestion, supports gut health, and promotes a feeling of fullness, which can help prevent overeating.

- **Weight Management**: Plant-based foods are often lower in calories yet filling, helping with healthy weight management.

Environmental Benefits of a Plant-Forward Diet

Beyond personal health, plant-based eating has a significant positive impact on the planet:

- **Lower Greenhouse Gas Emissions**: Plant-based foods have a lower carbon footprint compared to animal products, as they require less energy, water, and land to produce.

- **Reduces Deforestation**: Much of the world's deforestation is driven by the need for more land for livestock. By eating more plants, we help reduce the demand for new grazing land, thus preserving forests.

- **Less Water Usage**: Growing plants generally requires far less water than raising animals, which supports water conservation efforts.

Simple Ways to Start Eating More Plant-Based

1. **Choose One Plant-Based Meal a Day**: Try swapping one meal each day for a plant-based option. Start with something simple, like oatmeal with fruit for breakfast or a salad loaded with vegetables and legumes for lunch.

2. **Experiment with Meat Alternatives**: Enjoy new recipes with lentils, chickpeas, tofu, or tempeh as a protein source.

3. **Add More Vegetables to Your Plate**: Increase the portion of vegetables in each meal. You don't have to remove other foods entirely; just focus on adding more plants.

Embracing Local and Seasonal Eating

Eating locally and seasonally isn't just a fun way to explore new flavors; it's also one of the most effective ways to reduce the environmental impact of our diet.

Benefits of Local Eating

- **Reduces Carbon Emissions**: Local foods travel shorter distances, which means less fuel is used for transportation.
- **Supports the Local Economy**: Buying from local farmers helps strengthen the community and provides direct support to local businesses.
- **Fresher Produce**: Local fruits and vegetables are often fresher and tastier since they're harvested closer to their peak ripeness.

Why Seasonal Eating Matters

Seasonal eating means choosing foods that are naturally ready to harvest in your area at certain times of the year. It supports environmental sustainability because:

- **It Requires Less Energy**: Seasonal produce grows in harmony with natural conditions, requiring less artificial energy, like heating for greenhouses.
- **Reduces Food Waste**: Seasonal foods are usually more abundant, affordable, and less likely to spoil before reaching consumers, leading to less food waste.

Ways to Start Eating Locally and Seasonally

1. **Visit Farmers' Markets**: Local farmers' markets are a great place to find fresh, seasonal produce, often grown without excessive pesticides.
2. **Research Seasonal Produce**: Make a list of fruits and vegetables available in your region each season. Use it as a guide for meal planning.

3. **Join a Community Supported Agriculture (CSA) Program**: CSA programs allow you to receive regular deliveries of seasonal produce from local farms, often with variety and freshness unmatched by grocery stores.

Mindful Consumption: Reducing Food Waste

Approximately one-third of all food produced globally is wasted, which contributes to greenhouse gas emissions and squanders resources like water and energy. By making a few small adjustments, we can significantly reduce food waste.

Steps to Reduce Food Waste

- **Plan Meals**: Plan your meals for the week, which helps avoid impulse purchases and food that ends up unused.

- **Store Food Properly**: Many fruits and vegetables last longer if stored correctly. For example, refrigerating apples and carrots keeps them fresh for weeks.

- **Use "Scraps" Wisely**: Many vegetable scraps can be saved for soups, sauces, or even homemade vegetable broth.

- **Embrace Leftovers**: Leftovers can be a convenient, waste-free meal option. Try incorporating them into a new dish, like turning roast vegetables into a salad or pasta.

The Personal and Environmental Benefits of Reducing Food Waste

- **Reduces Greenhouse Gas Emissions**: When food waste decomposes in landfills, it releases methane, a potent greenhouse gas. By reducing waste, we help mitigate climate change.

- **Saves Money**: By buying only what you need and making use of leftovers, you can save significantly on grocery bills.

- **Fosters a Gratitude for Food**: Being mindful of waste fosters a deeper appreciation for food, from the farmers who grow it to the journey it takes to reach your plate.

Putting It All Together: Crafting a Sustainable Diet That Works for You

Creating a sustainable, health-supporting diet doesn't mean overhauling everything overnight. It's about gradually incorporating new habits and being intentional with each choice. Here's a step-by-step guide to get started:

1. **Set Small Goals**: Begin with one or two changes, like adding a plant-based meal or shopping at a farmers' market once a week.

2. **Experiment with Recipes**: Find joy in the process by trying new recipes and cooking techniques. Sustainable eating should be enjoyable, not restrictive.

3. **Reflect on Your Journey**: Track how you feel as you make these changes. Many people find that eco-friendly eating improves their energy, digestion, and overall mood.

4. **Stay Open to Growth**: Remember, sustainable eating is a journey, not a fixed destination. Continue to learn about new practices, experiment with seasonal foods, and evolve your diet over time.

Conclusion

Eating in a way that nourishes both your body and the planet can transform not only your health but also your relationship with food. Each choice—from selecting more plants to reducing food waste—has a positive impact that goes far beyond the dining table. As you continue on this journey, remember that sustainable eating is not about being perfect. It's about making choices that align with your values, benefit your well-being, and support the Earth.

CHAPTER 3: DETOXING YOUR HOME ENVIRONMENT

Our homes should be our ultimate sanctuaries—a place to feel safe, healthy, and renewed. Yet, many household items we encounter daily contain invisible chemicals that impact our health, even in small doses. From cleaning supplies to furniture and scented candles, common household products often release toxins into the air, affecting everything from respiratory health to sleep quality and long-term wellness.

In this chapter, we'll explore how to identify and reduce these hidden toxins, creating a clean, eco-friendly space that promotes well-being. By choosing natural, sustainable alternatives, you can transform your home into a truly safe haven for you, your loved ones, and the planet.

1. Unmasking Household Toxins: Where Are They Hiding?

Before diving into specific changes, it's important to understand the various sources of toxins in our homes and how they can impact our health. Many everyday products release volatile organic compounds (VOCs), tiny particles that easily become airborne, allowing us to inhale or absorb them through the skin.

Common Household Toxins

1. **Formaldehyde**: Found in pressed wood furniture, cabinets, and some fabrics, this VOC is linked to respiratory irritation and allergic reactions.

2. **Phthalates**: Present in synthetic fragrances, plastics, and cosmetics, these chemicals can disrupt hormones and may impact reproductive health.

3. **Triclosan**: Often found in antibacterial soaps and personal care products, triclosan has been associated with hormone disruption and may contribute to antibiotic resistance.

4. **Flame Retardants**: Used in furniture and electronics, flame retardants are linked to neurological and developmental concerns, especially in children.

5. **BPA and BPA Alternatives**: Common in plastic containers and canned food linings, BPA can leach into food and disrupt hormonal balance. Even "BPA-free" alternatives often contain similar compounds.

Understanding where these toxins are hiding helps us make informed choices, allowing us to begin the process of detoxifying our homes.

2. Cleaning With Care: Non-Toxic Alternatives For A Healthier Home

Household cleaners are a primary source of toxins, yet they're often marketed as essential for a clean, healthy home. Many conventional cleaners contain harsh chemicals that can irritate the skin, eyes, and respiratory tract, as well as damage the environment when they're washed down the drain.

Non-Toxic Cleaning Ingredients and Methods

- **Vinegar and Baking Soda**: This classic duo cleans effectively without harmful chemicals. Baking soda acts as a gentle abrasive, while vinegar dissolves dirt, kills bacteria, and neutralizes odors.
- **Lemon Juice**: Naturally acidic, lemon juice can cut through grease, remove stains, and leave surfaces smelling fresh.
- **Castile Soap**: This plant-based soap is gentle yet effective, suitable for a wide range of cleaning tasks, including dishes, countertops, and even laundry.
- **Essential Oils**: Tea tree, eucalyptus, and lavender essential oils have natural antimicrobial properties, making them excellent additions to homemade cleaners.

Homemade Cleaner Recipes

- **All-Purpose Spray**: Mix equal parts white vinegar and water, and add a few drops of tea tree oil for a natural disinfectant. Use on countertops, tiles, and other surfaces.
- **Bathroom Scrub**: Combine baking soda with castile soap until it forms a paste. Apply to bathroom surfaces with a sponge or brush, then rinse.
- **Window Cleaner**: Mix one part vinegar with one part

water, adding a few drops of lemon essential oil. Spray on glass and wipe with a lint-free cloth for a streak-free finish.

Additional Tips for a Non-Toxic Clean

1. **Ventilate While Cleaning**: Open windows or use fans while cleaning to help air out any lingering fumes.

2. **Declutter Regularly**: Keeping spaces organized and clutter-free reduces dust buildup, limiting exposure to dust-borne pollutants.

3. **Limit Use of Disinfectants**: Unless absolutely necessary, avoid overusing disinfectants. They can disrupt the natural microbiome of your home, which helps maintain a healthy immune system.

3. Choosing Non-Toxic Furnishings And Decor

Furniture, carpets, and textiles are other significant sources of toxins. Many new furnishings are treated with chemical preservatives or finishes that off-gas for months, sometimes years. By being selective about what we bring into our homes, we can reduce exposure to these chemicals and create a healthier living space.

Safer Furniture Choices

- **Opt for Solid Wood**: Choose furniture made from solid wood rather than pressed wood, which often contains formaldehyde and other toxic binders.

- **Look for VOC-Free Finishes**: Low or no-VOC finishes are available for furniture and paints, reducing airborne toxins in your home.

- **Prioritize Natural Materials**: Furniture made from materials like natural wood, metal, cotton, wool, and linen emit fewer chemicals than synthetic options.

Healthier Textiles and Flooring

- **Organic Cotton and Wool**: Look for bedding, towels, and other textiles made from organic fibers, as these are less likely to contain pesticides, synthetic dyes, and flame retardants.

- **Natural Fiber Rugs**: Rugs made from wool, jute, or cotton are safer options than synthetic carpets, which can release VOCs and microplastics.

- **Avoid Chemical Stain Repellents**: Stain repellents often contain perfluorinated chemicals (PFCs), which can disrupt hormones and linger in the environment for years. Opt for untreated fabrics or use natural protectants.

Reducing Dust and Particulates

Dust particles in the home often carry pollutants from furnishings, electronics, and other sources. To limit exposure:

1. **Use a HEPA Filter Vacuum**: Vacuum carpets and rugs weekly with a vacuum equipped with a HEPA filter to capture small particles.

2. **Dust with Damp Cloths**: A damp cloth captures dust better than dry dusting, which can release dust into the air.

3. **Avoid Wall-to-Wall Carpeting**: Carpeting can trap dust, dander, and allergens. Consider using area rugs that are easier to clean.

4. Improving Indoor Air Quality

Indoor air quality can significantly affect physical and mental health, especially for people with asthma, allergies, or chemical sensitivities. Besides choosing non-toxic materials, there are proactive ways to improve air quality naturally.

Natural Methods for Cleaner Indoor Air

1. **Ventilate Regularly**: Open windows daily, even in colder weather, to allow fresh air to circulate and flush out indoor pollutants.

2. **Invest in Houseplants**: Plants like spider plants, peace lilies, and English ivy naturally filter certain toxins from the air, contributing to cleaner indoor air.

3. **Use Activated Charcoal Air Filters**: Activated charcoal helps to absorb VOCs and odors, making it an eco-friendly option for maintaining fresh indoor air.

4. **Choose Beeswax or Soy Candles**: Regular paraffin candles can emit soot and toxins. Beeswax and soy candles burn cleanly, providing a natural way to add ambiance without polluting the air.

Air Purifier Options

For homes in areas with high outdoor pollution or for people with severe allergies, an air purifier with a HEPA filter can make a substantial difference. Look for purifiers that filter out allergens, smoke, and VOCs for a comprehensive air-cleaning effect.

5. Eliminating Synthetic Fragrances

Synthetic fragrances in products like air fresheners, candles, and personal care items contain chemicals that can disrupt hormones and contribute to respiratory problems. These scents are often marketed as fresh or clean but can introduce unnecessary toxins into your home.

Natural Alternatives for a Fresh-Smelling Home

- **Essential Oil Diffusers**: Diffusing essential oils like lavender, eucalyptus, or lemon offers a natural fragrance without the health risks associated with synthetic fragrances.

- **Simmer Pots**: Boil a pot of water with herbs, citrus slices, and spices to create a pleasant aroma in your home. It's a simple, natural way to refresh your space.

- **Herbal Sachets**: Place sachets filled with dried herbs like lavender or rosemary in closets, drawers, or other small spaces for a subtle, natural scent.

6. Detoxing Your Bedroom For Better Sleep

Since we spend around a third of our lives in our bedrooms, creating a toxin-free sleeping space is essential for improving sleep quality and overall health. By reducing toxins, you allow your body to rest and recover fully each night.

Steps for a Healthier Bedroom

1. **Choose a Non-Toxic Mattress**: Many mattresses contain flame retardants, synthetic foams, and adhesives that release VOCs. Opt for a mattress made from organic latex, wool, or cotton, which are free from these chemicals.

2. **Use Organic Bedding**: Choose sheets and pillowcases made from organic cotton or linen. These materials are breathable, chemical-free, and often softer than conventional textiles.

3. **Limit Electronics**: Electronics emit blue light and electromagnetic fields (EMFs), which can interfere with sleep quality. Keep phones, tablets, and TVs out of the bedroom or use "night mode" settings.

4. **Purify the Air**: Use an air purifier with a HEPA filter in your bedroom to maintain clean air while you sleep.

7. Reducing Plastic Use In The Home

Plastics are ubiquitous in modern homes, but they release harmful chemicals like BPA, phthalates, and microplastics, which can be absorbed by food and water or released into the air. Reducing plastic, especially in the kitchen, is a practical way to limit exposure to these chemicals.

Alternatives to Plastic

- **Glass Food Containers**: Store food in glass jars or containers instead of plastic. Glass doesn't leach chemicals into food and is reusable, durable, and eco-friendly.

- **Wooden Kitchen Utensils**: Plastic utensils can release microplastics, especially when exposed to heat. Switch to wood, bamboo, or stainless steel for a safer, longer-lasting option.

- **Natural Fiber Kitchen Sponges**: Synthetic sponges can shed microplastics. Opt for compostable sponges made from natural fibers like cotton or cellulose.

Conclusion

Detoxing your home environment is a powerful step toward a healthier, more balanced life. By reducing exposure to toxic chemicals, choosing eco-friendly alternatives, and implementing mindful cleaning practices, you create a home that supports well-being for you and your loved ones.

Remember, transforming your home doesn't have to happen overnight. Each small choice adds up, bringing you closer to a space that feels cleaner, safer, and more in harmony with nature. With every change, you're not only enhancing your health but also reducing your impact on the planet—creating a living environment that's truly sustainable in every sense.

CHAPTER 4: MINDFULNESS IN CONSUMPTION

In today's world, we're constantly surrounded by messages encouraging us to buy more, upgrade, and replace what we already have. The cycle of consumption can feel overwhelming and endless, often resulting in cluttered homes, financial strain, and unnecessary waste that harms the environment. Mindful consumption is a refreshing alternative —a way of living with intention, focusing on quality over quantity, and making choices that align with our values.

In this chapter, we'll explore the concept of mindful consumption and how it can help us lead simpler, healthier, and more meaningful lives. You'll learn practical strategies for reducing waste, making intentional purchases, and creating a balanced, clutter-free environment that fosters peace and purpose. Each choice you make in your daily life can be a step toward a sustainable future that benefits both you and the planet.

1. Understanding The Principles Of Mindful Consumption

Mindful consumption is about being aware of the impact of our choices, from the resources used to create an item to its journey from manufacturer to our home. This approach encourages us to consider not only the cost and convenience of each purchase but also its environmental and personal impact. By focusing on what we truly need and value, we can make more intentional, meaningful decisions.

Core Principles of Mindful Consumption

1. **Intentionality**: Asking yourself if a purchase truly aligns with your needs, values, and long-term goals.

2. **Awareness of Impact**: Recognizing the environmental, economic, and social impacts of what we consume.

3. **Quality Over Quantity**: Choosing well-made, durable items that will serve you over the long term.

4. **Appreciation and Gratitude**: Cultivating an appreciation for what we have and being mindful not to take resources for granted.

Mindful consumption is not about deprivation; it's about curating a lifestyle that aligns with your values, fostering a sense of fulfillment and purpose.

2. Reducing Waste: Practical Steps For Sustainable Living

Reducing waste is a core aspect of mindful consumption, benefiting both the planet and our homes by creating less clutter and lowering our environmental impact. With landfills overflowing and pollution on the rise, even small actions can make a significant difference.

Waste Reduction Strategies

- **The 5 Rs of Sustainability**: Refuse, Reduce, Reuse, Recycle, and Rot (Compost). These principles serve as a guide for making more sustainable choices and reducing waste at each step.
  - **Refuse**: Say no to items you don't need, like single-use plastic bags, flyers, or freebies.
  - **Reduce**: Limit the amount of new items you bring into your home by focusing on needs rather than wants.
  - **Reuse**: Opt for reusable items over disposable ones—use cloth bags, glass jars, and stainless-steel bottles.
  - **Recycle**: Properly sort recyclables, understanding local recycling guidelines to avoid contamination.
  - **Rot (Compost)**: Composting food scraps and organic waste is an excellent way to reduce landfill contributions and create nutrient-rich soil.
- **Adopt a Zero-Waste Mindset**: Aim to reduce waste as much as possible. Start small, like carrying a reusable water bottle and refusing plastic straws, and gradually expand to more impactful changes like shopping from bulk stores and minimizing packaging.

- **Repurpose and Upcycle**: Get creative with items you might otherwise throw away. Glass jars can be used for storage, old fabrics can become cleaning cloths, and cardboard can be composted or used for gardening.

3. Decluttering And Embracing Minimalism

Minimalism isn't about living with nothing; it's about removing the excess so that what remains truly adds value to your life. Clutter not only creates physical chaos but can also lead to stress, anxiety, and decision fatigue. By embracing minimalism and clearing out what doesn't serve us, we create space for what matters most.

Benefits of Minimalism

- **Reduces Stress**: A clutter-free space promotes calmness and mental clarity, creating a more relaxing environment.

- **Increases Focus**: By clearing away unnecessary items, you reduce distractions and can focus better on your tasks.

- **Promotes Mindful Living**: Minimalism encourages us to evaluate what we own and consider what we truly value.

Steps for a Mindful Decluttering Process

1. **Start Small**: Begin with one room, closet, or drawer at a time, rather than tackling the entire home at once.

2. **Sort Items**: Create piles for items to keep, donate, recycle, and discard. Ask yourself if each item is useful, brings joy, or holds sentimental value.

3. **Quality over Quantity**: When deciding what to keep, focus on well-made items that serve a purpose and align with your lifestyle.

4. **Regularly Reevaluate**: Minimalism is an ongoing process, not a one-time event. Periodically go through belongings to keep clutter at bay.

4. Choosing Quality Over Quantity

In a world where cheap, disposable products are the norm, choosing quality over quantity can feel like a revolutionary act. Quality items may have a higher upfront cost, but they often last longer, function better, and bring more satisfaction than their disposable counterparts. This approach not only saves money in the long run but also reduces waste by minimizing the need for replacements.

Benefits of Investing in Quality

- **Longevity**: High-quality items are built to last, reducing the need for frequent replacements.
- **Better Performance**: Well-made products often work better and provide a superior experience.
- **Reduced Environmental Impact**: Buying fewer, better-quality items leads to less waste and a smaller carbon footprint over time.

How to Choose Quality Items

1. **Research and Reviews**: Look for reputable brands and read reviews to ensure the product meets your needs.
2. **Look for Sustainable Certifications**: For items like clothing, electronics, or furniture, check for certifications that verify ethical and sustainable production, like Fair Trade, GOTS (Global Organic Textile Standard), or FSC (Forest Stewardship Council).
3. **Assess Materials and Craftsmanship**: Durable materials like stainless steel, organic cotton, and responsibly sourced wood are signs of a quality product.

Making the shift to quality items may take time, but it's a worthwhile investment in a sustainable, fulfilling lifestyle.

5. Shopping With Intention: A Guide To Mindful Purchases

Mindful consumption isn't about never buying anything new; it's about being intentional with each purchase. This approach helps prevent impulse buying, reduces waste, and ensures that every item serves a purpose in your life.

Tips for Shopping Mindfully

- **Pause Before Purchasing**: Before buying something, give yourself time to reflect. Ask yourself if it's a need, if it aligns with your values, and if it will genuinely add value to your life.

- **Make a List**: Whether shopping for groceries or personal items, lists help you stick to what you need and avoid unnecessary purchases.

- **Consider the Longevity**: Think about whether the item will be useful and enjoyable years down the line. Avoid items that will quickly wear out or go out of style.

- **Support Ethical Brands**: Seek out brands that prioritize sustainability, fair wages, and eco-friendly materials. By supporting responsible companies, you contribute to a better future.

Mindful shopping doesn't mean saying "no" to everything; it means saying "yes" to what truly matters.

6. Sustainable Habits For Daily Life

Beyond purchases, daily habits and routines can have a profound impact on consumption. By cultivating eco-friendly habits, we can live more sustainably without sacrificing convenience or comfort.

Daily Habits for a Mindful, Sustainable Lifestyle

- **Eat Mindfully**: Plan meals to reduce food waste, buy locally whenever possible, and opt for plant-based foods, which have a smaller environmental footprint.
- **Practice Energy Conservation**: Small habits like turning off lights when not in use, unplugging appliances, and choosing energy-efficient light bulbs add up to big energy savings over time.
- **Limit Water Use**: Take shorter showers, use low-flow fixtures, and fix leaks promptly to reduce water waste.
- **Reduce Packaging**: Bring reusable bags and containers when shopping, buy in bulk, and choose items with minimal or recyclable packaging.

Building New Habits with Ease

1. **Set Realistic Goals**: Start with one or two habits at a time to avoid feeling overwhelmed.
2. **Use Reminders**: Leave reminders for yourself, like keeping reusable bags in the car or setting a timer to limit shower time.
3. **Celebrate Progress**: Recognize your achievements, whether it's remembering to bring your reusable coffee cup or switching to energy-efficient light bulbs.

By creating sustainable routines, you'll make eco-friendly living a natural part of your lifestyle.

7. Cultivating Gratitude For What You Have

In a society that often emphasizes acquiring more, practicing gratitude for what we already have is a powerful act. Gratitude shifts the focus from what we lack to what we possess, fostering contentment and reducing the urge to consume unnecessarily.

Practicing Gratitude to Curb Excess Consumption

- **Reflect on Your Belongings**: Take time to appreciate the items that serve you well, from a favorite sweater to a comfortable chair. Acknowledging the value of these items can reduce the impulse to buy more.

- **Focus on Experiences Over Possessions**: Studies show that experiences bring more lasting happiness than material possessions. Invest in experiences that enrich your life, like spending time in nature, visiting museums, or sharing a meal with friends.

- **Keep a Gratitude Journal**: Regularly write down things you're grateful for—whether material items, relationships, or moments of joy. This practice fosters a mindset of abundance, reducing the urge to acquire more.

Gratitude is a simple yet transformative habit that can help shift your perspective on consumption.

Conclusion: The Rewards of Mindful Consumption

Mindful consumption is a powerful way to live intentionally, make a positive impact on the planet, and reduce unnecessary stress in your life. By focusing on what truly matters, embracing quality over quantity, and cultivating gratitude, you create a lifestyle that is rich in meaning and aligned with your values.

As you journey toward mindful consumption, remember that it's a gradual process. Each choice—whether it's refusing a plastic bag, selecting a durable product, or reflecting before a purchase—contributes to a more sustainable, fulfilling way of life. Embracing mindful consumption isn't about perfection; it's about progress, purpose, and creating a life that brings you joy and leaves a lighter footprint on the world.

By practicing mindful consumption, you not only free yourself from the clutter and stress of excess but also play a part in building a more sustainable future for all.

CHAPTER 5: NATURE THERAPY: THE HEALING POWER OF GREEN SPACES

In a world that often feels fast-paced and technology-driven, it's easy to become disconnected from nature. Yet, being in nature has profound and scientifically supported benefits for both mental and physical health. Nature therapy, also known as ecotherapy or green therapy, taps into these benefits, offering a way to reduce stress, boost mood, improve focus, and promote a sense of peace. This chapter will explore how to harness the power of nature to enhance well-being and incorporate green spaces into daily life, whether you live in a rural area, a city, or somewhere in between.

You'll learn about the science behind nature's healing effects, easy ways to include nature in your routine, and specific activities that can help you reconnect with the natural world. From forest bathing and gardening to simply spending time with houseplants, the opportunities for nature therapy are accessible to everyone, offering a pathway to a healthier, more balanced life.

1. The Science Of Nature Therapy: How Nature Heals

Recent research has shown that spending time in nature offers numerous health benefits, from reducing stress and anxiety to lowering blood pressure and strengthening the immune system. Exposure to natural elements, such as trees, water, and sunlight, triggers physiological responses that contribute to healing and relaxation. The science behind nature therapy provides compelling evidence of why spending time outdoors can have such a profound impact on well-being.

Key Health Benefits of Nature Exposure

- **Reduced Stress Levels**: Nature has been shown to lower levels of cortisol, the body's primary stress hormone. Spending even short periods of time outside can help the body shift into a state of relaxation, which promotes overall health.

- **Improved Focus and Cognitive Function**: Studies have found that spending time in nature improves attention span, memory, and problem-solving skills, particularly for those who experience "attention fatigue" from prolonged focus on screens and technology.

- **Boosted Immune System**: Exposure to sunlight increases vitamin D production, which plays a vital role in immune function. Additionally, compounds called phytoncides, released by trees and plants, are known to boost immunity and support overall health.

- **Enhanced Mood and Mental Health**: Time in nature has been associated with increased levels of happiness, improved mood, and reduced symptoms of depression and anxiety.

By understanding the science behind nature's benefits, we can intentionally use nature therapy as a tool to support health and mental clarity.

2. Bringing Nature Into Everyday Life

While some of us have easy access to forests, beaches, or parks, others may live in urban areas where natural spaces are limited. The good news is that even small doses of nature can make a difference. By finding creative ways to connect with nature in everyday life, you can experience many of its benefits no matter where you live.

Ideas for Incorporating Nature Daily

- **Morning Sunlight Exposure**: Spend a few minutes outside each morning, allowing natural light to reset your circadian rhythm and improve sleep quality.

- **Lunch Break Walks**: If possible, take a short walk outside during lunch or after work. Walking in a nearby park or tree-lined street can provide a mental refresh.

- **Create a Green Workspace**: Add a few plants to your workspace or set up your desk near a window with a view. Research shows that even a small amount of greenery can reduce stress and improve focus.

- **Listen to Nature Sounds**: If outdoor access is limited, consider using apps or recordings of nature sounds, like flowing water, birdsong, or gentle rain. These sounds can evoke the calming effects of nature.

These small changes can have an uplifting effect on your mood, making nature a consistent part of your day.

3. Exploring Forest Bathing (Shinrin-Yoku)

Originating in Japan, the practice of shinrin-yoku, or forest bathing, is the act of spending time immersed in a forest environment to promote relaxation and well-being. Forest bathing isn't about exercise or goal-setting; it's simply about being present in nature, using all your senses to connect with your surroundings. This practice has gained international popularity and is backed by studies showing its effectiveness in reducing stress, lowering blood pressure, and boosting mental health.

Steps to Practice Forest Bathing

1. **Find a Natural Area**: A forest is ideal, but any wooded area, park, or nature preserve can work for forest bathing.

2. **Turn Off Distractions**: Leave your phone in the car or turn it off to fully disconnect.

3. **Engage Your Senses**: Walk slowly, noticing the colors, textures, and smells around you. Listen to the rustle of leaves, the chirping of birds, or the wind.

4. **Breathe Deeply**: Take slow, mindful breaths. Phytoncides, compounds released by trees, can reduce stress and enhance relaxation.

5. **Take Your Time**: Forest bathing isn't rushed. Spend at least 20-30 minutes in nature, focusing on being present and observing without judgment.

Forest bathing is a simple yet profound way to slow down, reconnect with nature, and experience the healing power of green spaces.

4. The Healing Power Of Gardening

Gardening is a form of nature therapy that combines the benefits of physical activity, exposure to natural elements, and the rewarding experience of nurturing life. Whether it's a small windowsill herb garden, a backyard vegetable patch, or a few indoor plants, gardening provides a unique opportunity to connect with the earth and enjoy nature's therapeutic effects.

Health Benefits of Gardening

- **Physical Exercise**: Gardening involves various levels of physical activity, from digging and planting to weeding and harvesting. It's a low-impact workout that improves flexibility, strength, and coordination.

- **Mental Health Boost**: Tending to plants and watching them grow brings a sense of accomplishment and purpose, which can reduce symptoms of depression and anxiety.

- **Exposure to Sunlight and Fresh Air**: Spending time outdoors in the garden promotes vitamin D production and increases oxygen intake, supporting overall health and immunity.

- **Mindfulness and Stress Reduction**: Gardening encourages mindfulness by focusing on simple, repetitive tasks. The act of caring for plants can create a sense of calm and focus, reducing mental clutter.

Ways to Get Started with Gardening

1. **Start Small**: If you're new to gardening, start with a few easy-to-grow plants, such as herbs or leafy greens.

2. **Choose Native Plants**: Native plants are adapted to the local climate and require less water and maintenance, making them an eco-friendly choice.

3. **Engage the Senses**: Choose plants that stimulate the

senses, such as fragrant herbs like lavender, colorful flowers, or textured foliage.

4. **Practice Patience**: Gardening is a gradual process that teaches patience and acceptance of nature's cycles. Embrace the journey as you watch your plants grow.

Gardening offers a hands-on way to experience the benefits of nature therapy, and it's an activity that anyone can enjoy, regardless of space or skill level.

5. Bringing Nature Indoors: Houseplants And Indoor Green Spaces

For those with limited access to outdoor green spaces, houseplants can bring the benefits of nature indoors. Studies show that having plants in your home can improve indoor air quality, reduce stress, and even increase productivity. Plants create a soothing atmosphere and can help you feel more connected to nature, even indoors.

Benefits of Indoor Plants

- **Improved Air Quality**: Some houseplants, like spider plants, peace lilies, and snake plants, help filter indoor pollutants and increase oxygen levels.

- **Reduced Stress and Anxiety**: Simply having greenery in your home can reduce stress levels, promote relaxation, and improve mood.

- **Enhanced Focus and Productivity**: Houseplants have been shown to boost concentration and productivity, making them a great addition to workspaces.

- **Boosted Humidity**: Plants release moisture into the air, which can be beneficial for skin, respiratory health, and overall indoor comfort.

Tips for Creating an Indoor Green Space

1. **Choose Low-Maintenance Plants**: Start with easy-care plants like pothos, ZZ plants, or snake plants, which are resilient and don't require frequent watering.

2. **Arrange by Natural Light**: Place plants near windows where they can receive natural light. Some plants prefer indirect light, while others thrive in bright, direct light.

3. **Incorporate Plants into Decor**: Use plant stands, hanging pots, or wall-mounted planters to incorporate

greenery into your home's design.

4. **Add a Water Element**: For an extra touch of nature, consider adding a small indoor water feature, such as a tabletop fountain, which can promote relaxation and mimic the sound of flowing water.

Bringing nature indoors allows you to enjoy the benefits of green spaces year-round, regardless of the weather or your location.

6. Nature-Based Activities For Mental Health

Beyond gardening and forest bathing, there are numerous activities that leverage nature's calming effects to support mental health. Nature-based activities encourage mindfulness, foster a sense of wonder, and provide opportunities to disconnect from the stresses of daily life.

Effective Nature-Based Activities

- **Mindful Walking in Nature**: Walking in nature with mindfulness—paying attention to the sights, sounds, and smells around you—promotes relaxation and focus. Unlike regular exercise, mindful walking is slow and deliberate, encouraging you to be present in each step.

- **Outdoor Yoga and Meditation**: Practicing yoga or meditation outdoors enhances its calming effects by adding the natural elements of sunlight, fresh air, and natural sounds.

- **Birdwatching or Wildlife Observation**: Observing animals in their natural habitats fosters patience and wonder, helping you feel more connected to the ecosystem around you.

- **Beach or River Stone Collecting**: Many people find it therapeutic to collect stones, shells, or other natural objects. The process of gathering and appreciating these items encourages mindfulness and a sense of connection to the environment.

These activities can be adapted to various levels of mobility and access, making them suitable for everyone, from children to seniors.

Conclusion: Embracing Nature Therapy for a Balanced Life

Nature therapy offers a unique and accessible way to support both physical health and mental well-being. Whether it's through gardening, spending time in a forest, adding houseplants to your home, or simply taking mindful walks, connecting with nature brings balance, peace, and healing into our lives. Each interaction with nature strengthens our bond with the environment, reminding us of our place in the natural world.

By making nature a part of your daily routine, you can experience its transformative benefits and enjoy a renewed sense of harmony with the world around you. Embrace the opportunities for nature therapy that suit your lifestyle, and watch as the healing power of green spaces enriches your life, one step at a time.

CHAPTER 6: SUSTAINABLE MOVEMENT AND PHYSICAL WELL-BEING

In an era of gym memberships, high-tech workout gear, and fitness apps, it's easy to overlook the environmental impact of our exercise habits. Sustainable movement focuses on physical activity that respects the environment, aligns with nature, and supports our overall well-being. Whether it's choosing eco-friendly gear, exercising outdoors, or commuting by bike, sustainable movement connects us to our surroundings, encourages mindfulness, and benefits both our health and the planet.

In this chapter, we'll explore how to make exercise more sustainable by embracing low-impact activities, selecting eco-friendly gear, and reconnecting with nature through outdoor workouts. With each step, you'll discover how movement can nurture both your body and the Earth, making physical fitness an integral part of a balanced, green lifestyle.

1. Embracing The Health And Environmental Benefits Of Outdoor Exercise

One of the simplest ways to incorporate sustainability into physical fitness is to move your exercise outdoors. The natural environment offers countless benefits, from fresh air and sunlight to opportunities for mindfulness. Plus, outdoor exercise reduces the need for energy-consuming gym equipment, contributing to a lower carbon footprint.

Health Benefits of Outdoor Exercise

- **Improved Mental Health**: Exercising in nature can reduce symptoms of anxiety and depression, improve mood, and increase feelings of well-being. Studies show that "green exercise" stimulates endorphin release, enhancing happiness and stress relief.

- **Increased Vitamin D**: Sunlight exposure during outdoor exercise helps the body produce vitamin D, a nutrient essential for bone health, immune function, and mood regulation.

- **Enhanced Cardiovascular Health**: Walking, running, cycling, and other outdoor exercises help improve heart health, reduce blood pressure, and boost circulation.

- **Greater Variety and Flexibility**: Outdoor exercise is versatile, offering activities for all fitness levels and preferences, from trail running to yoga in the park.

Environmental Benefits of Outdoor Workouts

- **Lower Carbon Footprint**: Exercising outdoors reduces reliance on powered gym equipment and minimizes the energy consumption associated with indoor workouts.

- **Reduced Plastic and Waste**: By minimizing the use of

single-use water bottles, disposable wipes, and other gym products, outdoor exercise creates less waste.

- **Connection with Nature**: Outdoor movement fosters an appreciation for the natural environment, encouraging people to protect and preserve it for future generations.

Whether it's a hike through the woods, a run on the beach, or a bike ride through the city, outdoor exercise offers a sustainable way to move that supports both personal and planetary health.

2. Sustainable Commuting: Walking, Biking, And Active Transportation

One of the most effective ways to integrate sustainable movement into daily life is through active transportation —walking, biking, or using other forms of human-powered transport. These forms of commuting not only reduce emissions but also promote physical well-being, save money, and encourage mindfulness.

Benefits of Active Transportation

- **Reduced Carbon Emissions**: Choosing to walk or bike instead of driving reduces greenhouse gas emissions, contributing to cleaner air and a healthier environment.

- **Improved Physical Fitness**: Active transportation integrates movement into your daily routine, helping you reach fitness goals without additional time or effort.

- **Cost Savings**: Walking or biking instead of driving can save on fuel, car maintenance, and parking costs.

- **Mental Clarity and Focus**: Active commuting helps clear the mind, reduce stress, and boost mental focus, making it an excellent way to start and end the workday.

Practical Tips for Sustainable Commuting

1. **Invest in a Quality Bike**: A well-maintained, durable bike can provide years of eco-friendly transportation. Consider purchasing a used or refurbished bike to reduce demand for new materials.

2. **Use Public Transportation When Possible**: Combining public transit with walking or biking is an effective way to reduce your carbon footprint.

3. **Plan Safe Routes**: Use bike lanes, sidewalks, and safe crossings to make commuting by foot or bike more convenient and enjoyable.

4. **Prioritize Walking for Short Distances**: For trips less than a mile, consider walking rather than driving. It's a simple way to get moving and support sustainability.

Active transportation transforms your commute into a productive, health-promoting habit that aligns with eco-friendly values.

3. Eco-Friendly Fitness Gear: Choosing Sustainable Options

The fitness industry produces a significant amount of waste, from plastic water bottles and synthetic workout clothes to disposable equipment. Choosing sustainable gear can reduce waste, minimize your environmental impact, and support brands that prioritize ethical practices.

Tips for Selecting Eco-Friendly Fitness Gear

- **Opt for Natural Fabrics**: Look for workout clothes made from organic cotton, bamboo, or recycled materials. Natural fibers are often more breathable, reducing odor and the need for frequent washing.

- **Invest in Durable Equipment**: High-quality, long-lasting equipment, like yoga mats, resistance bands, and dumbbells, reduces the need for frequent replacements. Avoid cheaply made items that wear out quickly.

- **Use a Reusable Water Bottle**: A reusable bottle made from stainless steel or glass reduces plastic waste and keeps water cool throughout your workout.

- **Seek Out Sustainable Brands**: Many fitness brands are committed to sustainable practices, using recycled materials, eco-friendly dyes, and ethical labor. Look for brands with certifications like Fair Trade, GOTS (Global Organic Textile Standard), or OEKO-TEX.

Eco-Friendly Workout Accessories

1. **Yoga Mats**: Choose mats made from natural rubber, cork, or recycled materials. Avoid PVC mats, which are non-biodegradable and may release harmful chemicals.

2. **Tote Bags**: Use a sustainable tote bag to carry gym

essentials, rather than disposable plastic or paper bags.

3. **Fitness Apparel**: Look for clothes made from recycled polyester or other sustainable fabrics. Brands like Patagonia and prAna offer eco-conscious options.

Choosing eco-friendly gear supports sustainable practices, helps reduce landfill waste, and ensures you're investing in quality items that will last.

4. Mindful And Low-Impact Exercise Practices

Not all exercise has to be high-impact or intense to be effective. Low-impact exercise, such as yoga, pilates, and tai chi, offers gentle, sustainable ways to improve flexibility, balance, and core strength without putting excess strain on the body. These forms of movement also encourage mindfulness, a practice that benefits both mental and physical health.

Benefits of Low-Impact Exercise

- **Reduces Injury Risk**: Low-impact exercises are gentle on the joints and reduce the likelihood of injury, making them suitable for all ages and fitness levels.

- **Promotes Mindfulness**: Many low-impact exercises emphasize breath control, body awareness, and mental focus, supporting relaxation and reducing stress.

- **Increases Flexibility and Balance**: Practices like yoga and tai chi improve flexibility, balance, and posture, which can enhance overall mobility.

- **Supports Long-Term Sustainability**: Low-impact exercise can be sustained over a lifetime, making it a valuable addition to any fitness routine.

Incorporating Low-Impact Movement into Daily Life

1. **Try Gentle Yoga or Pilates**: These forms of exercise build strength and flexibility without the need for heavy equipment or high-intensity movements.

2. **Explore Tai Chi or Qi Gong**: Rooted in ancient practices, these exercises combine gentle movement with deep breathing and are often practiced outdoors.

3. **Use Body Weight for Resistance**: Simple movements like squats, lunges, and planks use your body weight for resistance, making them accessible and equipment-free.

Low-impact exercise is ideal for maintaining physical health in a sustainable, mindful way.

5. Outdoor Group Activities: Building Community And Connection

Group activities foster a sense of community and provide motivation, helping people stay engaged and accountable to their fitness goals. Outdoor group activities, like hiking clubs, beach volleyball, and outdoor fitness classes, provide these benefits while reducing the environmental impact of indoor, energy-consuming gyms.

Benefits of Outdoor Group Fitness

- **Increased Motivation**: Group activities provide accountability and encouragement, making it easier to stay committed.

- **Social Connection**: Exercising with others builds community, fosters friendships, and reduces feelings of isolation.

- **Lower Environmental Impact**: Outdoor activities don't require the energy consumption associated with gym equipment and facilities.

- **Exposure to Fresh Air and Sunlight**: Exercising outdoors offers natural light and fresh air, enhancing mood and energy levels.

Ideas for Eco-Friendly Group Activities

1. **Join a Hiking or Walking Club**: Local hiking and walking groups provide a low-cost, eco-friendly way to stay active, explore nature, and meet new people.

2. **Outdoor Yoga or Fitness Classes**: Many parks and recreation areas offer outdoor classes. Look for yoga, boot camps, or fitness meetups in your area.

3. **Organize a Community Cleanup Workout**: Combine exercise with environmental action by organizing a group litter cleanup in a local park or beach. It's a

meaningful way to give back while staying active.

By participating in group outdoor activities, you build connections and support eco-friendly movement in your community.

6. Practicing Environmental Mindfulness During Exercise

Sustainable movement goes beyond the activities themselves; it also includes being mindful of our environmental impact during workouts. Practicing eco-conscious habits, from limiting waste to respecting nature, allows us to exercise in a way that honors the planet.

Eco-Friendly Exercise Habits

- **Leave No Trace**: When exercising outdoors, follow Leave No Trace principles—take all waste with you, avoid disturbing wildlife, and stay on designated trails.

- **Avoid Single-Use Plastics**: Bring reusable water bottles, containers, and towels, reducing reliance on disposable items.

- **Support Green Spaces**: Many parks and natural areas rely on donations and volunteer support. Consider donating or participating in conservation efforts.

- **Carpool or Use Public Transportation**: For group events or classes, carpool with friends or use public transit to reduce emissions.

Being environmentally mindful during exercise allows us to protect the spaces we enjoy and ensure that they remain available for future generations.

Conclusion: Sustainable Movement for Lifelong Health and Planetary Well-being

Sustainable movement aligns personal health with environmental stewardship, offering a holistic approach to physical fitness. By embracing outdoor exercise, choosing eco-friendly gear, practicing low-impact activities, and engaging in mindful, eco-conscious habits, you contribute to a healthier planet while nurturing your own body and mind.

Remember that sustainable movement is about creating a balanced approach that works for you. Whether it's a daily walk, a weekend hike, or a low-impact yoga session, each movement choice connects you to the Earth and supports your well-being. Embrace sustainable movement as a lifelong practice, one that fosters physical health, environmental awareness, and a deep appreciation for the natural world.

CHAPTER 7: RESTORATIVE LIVING: SLEEP, REST, AND ECO-FRIENDLY HABITS

In our fast-paced, always-connected world, sleep and rest often take a backseat to daily demands and busy schedules. Yet, adequate sleep and rest are essential for maintaining physical and mental health, balancing hormones, and strengthening immunity. In this chapter, we'll explore how to cultivate restorative living by focusing on sleep hygiene, eco-friendly sleep environments, and daily habits that promote deep rest and relaxation.

Restorative living isn't just about sleep; it's about creating a balanced lifestyle that values rest as much as productivity. By adopting eco-friendly practices, you'll create a sanctuary that supports a peaceful mind, a healthy body, and a more sustainable approach to life.

1. The Importance Of Sleep For Health And Well-Being

Sleep is a fundamental aspect of human health, yet it's often one of the first things we sacrifice when life gets busy. Poor sleep can lead to a range of health issues, including weakened immunity, poor mental health, and reduced cognitive performance. Quality sleep is essential for restoring the body, processing memories, and maintaining hormonal balance.

Key Health Benefits of Quality Sleep

- **Immune System Support**: Sleep is critical for immune function. During sleep, the body produces cytokines, proteins that help combat infection, inflammation, and stress.

- **Enhanced Cognitive Function**: Sleep allows the brain to process information, consolidate memories, and improve focus and creativity.

- **Emotional Well-Being**: Restorative sleep plays a vital role in regulating mood and reducing stress. Studies have shown that sleep-deprived individuals are more prone to anxiety, irritability, and depression.

- **Physical Recovery**: During deep sleep stages, the body repairs tissues, builds muscle, and releases growth hormones that are essential for recovery.

Understanding the importance of sleep underscores why investing in good sleep hygiene and an eco-friendly sleep environment is essential for a balanced, healthy life.

2. Creating An Eco-Friendly Bedroom For Restful Sleep

The bedroom should be a sanctuary for rest, free from environmental toxins and distractions. By choosing sustainable, non-toxic materials for your sleep environment, you'll reduce exposure to harmful chemicals and create a space that encourages restful, uninterrupted sleep.

Eco-Friendly Bedroom Essentials

1. **Organic Mattresses and Bedding**: Many mattresses contain flame retardants and synthetic materials that can release harmful VOCs. Choosing an organic mattress made from natural latex, organic cotton, or wool reduces exposure to these toxins.

2. **Natural Fiber Sheets and Blankets**: Opt for bedding made from organic cotton, linen, or bamboo, which are hypoallergenic, breathable, and free from pesticides and synthetic dyes.

3. **Air-Purifying Plants**: Certain plants, like snake plants, peace lilies, and aloe vera, help filter indoor air, improving air quality and promoting relaxation.

4. **Non-Toxic Paints and Finishes**: Many conventional paints contain VOCs, which can release harmful chemicals for years after application. Look for low-VOC or zero-VOC paints to maintain indoor air quality.

Additional Tips for a Restful, Eco-Friendly Bedroom

- **Use Blackout Curtains**: Exposure to artificial light during sleep can disrupt the circadian rhythm. Blackout curtains help create a dark environment, enhancing sleep quality.

- **Limit Electronics in the Bedroom**: Electronics emit blue light and electromagnetic fields (EMFs), which can interfere with sleep. Keep phones, tablets, and other devices out of the bedroom or switch them to "night mode" to reduce exposure.

- **Add a Natural Sound Machine**: For those who benefit from white noise, choose a sound machine that mimics natural sounds, such as rainfall, ocean waves, or birdsong. These sounds can enhance relaxation without adding unnecessary technology to the room.

An eco-friendly bedroom supports not only restful sleep but also a healthier environment by reducing exposure to synthetic chemicals and promoting clean air quality.

3. Sustainable Sleep Hygiene Practices

Good sleep hygiene involves establishing routines and behaviors that prepare the body and mind for restful sleep. Incorporating sustainable practices into your sleep routine can enhance relaxation and make winding down an enjoyable, eco-friendly experience.

Key Elements of Sustainable Sleep Hygiene

- **Establish a Consistent Sleep Schedule**: Going to bed and waking up at the same time each day reinforces your body's internal clock, making it easier to fall asleep and wake up naturally.

- **Limit Exposure to Artificial Light Before Bed**: Artificial light, particularly blue light from screens, can suppress melatonin production. Try dimming lights, using "night mode" on screens, or avoiding devices at least an hour before bed.

- **Create a Pre-Bed Relaxation Routine**: Engage in calming activities such as reading, meditating, or taking a warm bath. Opt for eco-friendly candles or essential oil diffusers to add a soothing ambiance.

- **Avoid Heavy Meals and Caffeine Late in the Day**: Food and caffeine can interfere with the body's natural sleep processes. Choose lighter, caffeine-free alternatives like herbal teas or warm water with lemon in the evening.

By practicing good sleep hygiene with an eco-conscious approach, you'll support a healthier lifestyle and improve the quality of your sleep.

4. Eco-Friendly Sleep Products For A Sustainable Bedtime Routine

Sustainable sleep products are designed with both the user and the environment in mind. These products are made from natural materials, free from harmful chemicals, and often have a lower environmental impact.

Recommended Eco-Friendly Sleep Products

1. **Natural Fiber Pajamas**: Choose sleepwear made from organic cotton, bamboo, or linen, which are soft, breathable, and free from synthetic fibers that can disrupt temperature regulation.

2. **Recycled or Organic Cotton Blankets**: Sustainable blankets and throws made from organic or recycled fibers offer warmth without the environmental toll of conventional textiles.

3. **Eco-Friendly Sleep Masks**: For those who sleep better in complete darkness, a sleep mask made from organic cotton or bamboo provides comfort without the synthetic materials.

4. **Herbal Sleep Aids**: Herbal teas like chamomile, valerian root, or lavender can help relax the mind and prepare the body for sleep. Opt for organic, sustainably sourced options to support both your health and the environment.

Natural Sleep-Inducing Scents

Certain scents, like lavender, chamomile, and sandalwood, are known for their calming effects. You can incorporate these scents into your bedtime routine by using:

- **Essential Oil Diffusers**: Add a few drops of lavender or chamomile oil to a diffuser for a natural, calming scent that promotes relaxation.

- **Pillow Sprays**: Look for organic pillow sprays made with essential oils to create a soothing environment as you settle in for the night.
- **Herbal Sachets**: Place a sachet filled with dried lavender or chamomile under your pillow for a gentle, natural aroma.

These eco-friendly products and scents contribute to a peaceful, sustainable sleep routine that aligns with restorative living.

5. The Role Of Rest And Relaxation In Sustainable Living

Restorative living goes beyond sleep—it includes all forms of rest and relaxation that recharge the body and mind. In our culture of constant productivity, intentionally prioritizing rest is a radical act that supports long-term health and happiness.

Health Benefits of Regular Rest and Relaxation

- **Reduced Stress Levels**: Intentional relaxation lowers cortisol levels, helping to prevent chronic stress and its related health issues.

- **Improved Focus and Productivity**: Regular breaks and moments of rest improve mental clarity, focus, and creativity, making us more effective in our daily tasks.

- **Better Emotional Health**: Relaxation practices foster resilience, helping us manage difficult emotions and reducing symptoms of anxiety and depression.

- **Enhanced Immune Function**: Rest allows the body to recharge, strengthening immunity and reducing vulnerability to illness.

By making time for rest, you support a balanced, fulfilling lifestyle that aligns with the principles of sustainability and self-care.

6. Mindfulness And Meditation As Restorative Practices

Mindfulness and meditation are powerful tools for relaxation and self-awareness. Practicing these techniques regularly reduces stress, improves sleep, and enhances well-being. Meditation encourages present-moment awareness, while mindfulness helps us tune into our environment, our bodies, and our emotions with greater clarity.

Simple Mindfulness Techniques for Daily Life

1. **Mindful Breathing**: Take a few minutes each day to focus on your breath, inhaling and exhaling slowly. This practice calms the mind and encourages a state of relaxation.

2. **Body Scan**: Lie down or sit comfortably and mentally scan each part of your body, starting from your toes and working up to your head. Release any tension as you focus on each area.

3. **Guided Meditation**: Use a meditation app or recording to follow a guided session that promotes relaxation. Many guided meditations are designed to reduce stress, improve focus, or prepare the mind for sleep.

4. **Nature Meditation**: Spend a few moments in nature, observing your surroundings without judgment. Focus on the sounds, smells, and sights around you, allowing your mind to quiet and relax.

Mindfulness practices not only improve rest and relaxation but also foster a deeper connection to the present moment, promoting a more balanced and intentional lifestyle.

7. Daily Habits To Promote Restorative Living

Incorporating rest into daily life doesn't require major changes; simple habits can make a big difference. By being intentional with our time and prioritizing activities that bring joy and relaxation, we create a lifestyle that naturally supports rest and well-being.

Daily Habits for Restorative Living

- **Take Short Breaks Throughout the Day**: Regular breaks prevent burnout, improve productivity, and reduce stress. Use these moments to stretch, breathe deeply, or take a quick walk outside.

- **Limit Screen Time Before Bed**: Excessive screen time can lead to digital eye strain, mental fatigue, and difficulty sleeping. Set boundaries to reduce screen time, especially before bed.

- **Create a Relaxing Evening Routine**: Wind down each evening with relaxing activities like reading, journaling, or gentle stretching.

- **Practice Gratitude**: Each day, take a moment to reflect on something you're grateful for. This practice promotes positivity, reduces stress, and supports emotional well-being.

By integrating these simple habits into your routine, you create a lifestyle that values and encourages restorative living.

Conclusion: Embracing Restorative Living for Sustainable Health and Well-Being

Restorative living is an essential component of a balanced, sustainable lifestyle. By prioritizing sleep, creating an eco-friendly sleep environment, and adopting daily habits that support rest, we foster a state of well-being that is both healthful and harmonious with nature.

As you incorporate these principles into your life, remember that rest and relaxation are not indulgences—they are necessities. When we invest in restorative living, we are better equipped to handle life's challenges, support those around us, and contribute to a more sustainable future. Embrace rest as an essential part of your journey toward well-being, allowing it to renew your mind, restore your body, and nurture your spirit.

CHAPTER 8: REDUCING ENVIRONMENTAL STRESSORS

Our surroundings profoundly impact our health, well-being, and mood. While we might think of stress as being primarily psychological, many stressors come from our environment. Noise pollution, artificial lighting, electromagnetic fields (EMFs), and even the air quality in our homes can contribute to mental and physical strain. Reducing these environmental stressors is essential for creating a balanced, health-promoting living space that supports relaxation, productivity, and peace of mind.

In this chapter, we'll explore the hidden stressors in our daily environments and learn practical ways to minimize them. By creating a low-stress environment, we can foster a lifestyle that's healthier, more mindful, and more aligned with sustainable living.

1. Understanding Environmental Stressors And Their Impact On Health

Environmental stressors are external factors that can affect our well-being and mood. These stressors range from noise and air quality to lighting and technology, impacting everything from our physical health to our mental clarity and energy levels.

Key Environmental Stressors

- **Noise Pollution**: Traffic, construction, and even household appliances contribute to noise pollution, which can increase stress, disrupt sleep, and reduce focus.

- **Poor Air Quality**: Indoor pollutants, including dust, VOCs (volatile organic compounds), and mold, can cause respiratory issues, fatigue, and exacerbate allergies.

- **Electromagnetic Fields (EMFs)**: EMFs from Wi-Fi routers, smartphones, and electronic devices are believed to impact sleep quality and may contribute to stress and fatigue.

- **Artificial Lighting**: Exposure to artificial light, particularly blue light, can interfere with sleep patterns, reduce melatonin production, and lead to digital eye strain.

Recognizing these stressors allows us to make informed changes that promote a healthier, less stressful living environment.

2. Minimizing Noise Pollution For A Calmer Home

Noise pollution is a major source of stress in modern life, impacting sleep, concentration, and overall well-being. Constant noise can elevate cortisol levels, the body's primary stress hormone, and lead to sleep disturbances that negatively affect health. Reducing noise pollution creates a quieter, more peaceful environment that promotes relaxation and focus.

Practical Tips to Reduce Noise Pollution

1. **Soundproof Key Areas**: If you live in a noisy area, consider soundproofing essential rooms, like bedrooms, with thick curtains, rugs, and door seals to block outside noise.

2. **Use White Noise Machines**: White noise machines or apps can mask unwanted noise and create a more consistent, soothing background sound that aids sleep and focus.

3. **Incorporate Natural Noise Barriers**: Place indoor plants near windows or invest in a water feature, like a small fountain, to create pleasant, natural sounds that help mask intrusive noise.

4. **Designate Quiet Zones**: Designate certain areas of the home as "quiet zones" for reading, meditation, or other relaxing activities, free from loud appliances and electronics.

Reducing noise pollution helps foster a calm atmosphere that's conducive to relaxation, concentration, and mental well-being.

3. Improving Indoor Air Quality For Better Health

Indoor air quality is crucial to our health, as we spend a significant amount of time indoors. Common indoor pollutants like dust, VOCs, mold, and pet dander can lead to respiratory issues, allergies, and fatigue. Improving air quality creates a cleaner, healthier living environment that supports lung health and enhances overall well-being.

Steps to Improve Indoor Air Quality

- **Use an Air Purifier**: High-quality air purifiers with HEPA filters capture dust, pollen, pet dander, and other airborne particles, reducing allergens and pollutants in the air.

- **Ventilate Regularly**: Open windows daily to let fresh air circulate and reduce the buildup of indoor pollutants.

- **Control Humidity**: Use a dehumidifier to maintain ideal humidity levels (30-50%), as excessive moisture promotes mold growth and dust mites.

- **Incorporate Air-Purifying Plants**: Plants like peace lilies, spider plants, and Boston ferns are known to filter certain pollutants, improving air quality naturally.

Improving indoor air quality doesn't just make your home feel fresher—it also reduces the risk of respiratory issues, improves sleep quality, and promotes overall health.

4. Limiting Exposure To Electromagnetic Fields (Emfs)

Electromagnetic fields (EMFs) are emitted by electronic devices, Wi-Fi routers, cell towers, and household appliances. Although research is ongoing, some studies suggest that long-term exposure to high EMF levels may impact sleep, contribute to stress, and affect overall health. Taking steps to reduce EMF exposure can create a more restful, low-stress environment.

Practical Tips to Reduce EMF Exposure

1. **Create an EMF-Free Bedroom**: Keep electronic devices out of the bedroom or place them at least several feet away from the bed to reduce EMF exposure during sleep.

2. **Turn Off Wi-Fi at Night**: When not in use, especially overnight, switch off Wi-Fi routers to reduce EMF exposure in the home.

3. **Opt for Wired Connections**: When possible, use wired internet connections instead of Wi-Fi, as this reduces the level of EMFs in your space.

4. **Use Airplane Mode on Devices**: If you keep your phone in the bedroom or carry it frequently, switch it to airplane mode when not in use to reduce EMF exposure.

Taking steps to reduce EMF exposure may support better sleep, reduce stress, and create a healthier environment.

5. Reducing Blue Light And Artificial Lighting In The Home

Exposure to artificial light, particularly blue light from screens, can disrupt our circadian rhythm and interfere with sleep. Blue light suppresses melatonin production, the hormone responsible for sleep regulation, making it difficult to fall asleep at night. By limiting blue light exposure and using natural lighting, you can support better sleep and reduce digital eye strain.

Ways to Manage Artificial and Blue Light Exposure

- **Use Warm, Low-Intensity Lighting in the Evening**: Opt for warm, dim lighting in the evening to help the body prepare for sleep. LED bulbs with lower blue light emissions are ideal for this purpose.

- **Limit Screen Time Before Bed**: Avoid screens, such as phones, tablets, and computers, at least an hour before bedtime to reduce blue light exposure.

- **Invest in Blue Light Filters**: Use blue light filtering glasses or software to minimize blue light exposure if you need to use screens in the evening.

- **Maximize Natural Light During the Day**: Spend time in natural light during the day, as exposure to natural sunlight helps regulate melatonin production and maintains a healthy circadian rhythm.

Reducing blue light exposure and maximizing natural light can enhance sleep quality, reduce eye strain, and improve mood and productivity.

6. Managing Temperature For Optimal Comfort And Sleep

The temperature of your environment has a significant impact on comfort, sleep quality, and stress levels. A cool, consistent temperature supports restful sleep and reduces the likelihood of night sweats and discomfort. Setting up an optimal temperature in your home, especially in the bedroom, can help create a more restful and comfortable space.

Tips for Managing Indoor Temperature

- **Maintain a Cool Bedroom**: Aim to keep your bedroom temperature between 60-67°F (15-19°C), as this range is considered optimal for restful sleep.

- **Use Natural Ventilation**: During cooler seasons, open windows to allow fresh air in and maintain a comfortable indoor temperature without relying on air conditioning.

- **Choose Breathable Bedding**: Opt for natural, breathable materials like cotton or linen for bedding, as they help regulate body temperature and prevent overheating.

- **Invest in a Programmable Thermostat**: A programmable thermostat can automatically adjust temperature settings throughout the day, creating a comfortable environment while saving energy.

Maintaining an ideal indoor temperature not only improves sleep quality but also contributes to a more energy-efficient, eco-friendly home.

7. Reducing Clutter For A Low-Stress Environment

Clutter creates visual and mental chaos, contributing to feelings of stress, anxiety, and overwhelm. By reducing clutter, you create a calming, organized space that promotes relaxation, productivity, and peace of mind. Decluttering is not only beneficial for mental well-being but also aligns with sustainable practices by encouraging mindful consumption and reducing waste.

Strategies for Decluttering and Organizing

- **Adopt a "One In, One Out" Rule**: For every new item you bring into your home, remove or donate an item to prevent clutter accumulation.

- **Create Designated Spaces**: Assign specific places for items, ensuring that everything has a home, making it easier to keep spaces organized.

- **Use Storage Solutions Wisely**: Utilize storage options like baskets, bins, and shelves to keep items out of sight and create a cleaner, more open space.

- **Declutter Regularly**: Periodically go through your belongings to assess what you truly need and use. Donate, recycle, or discard items that no longer serve a purpose.

Reducing clutter fosters a sense of calm, increases focus, and makes your home a more pleasant and functional space.

8. Creating A Calming And Balanced Atmosphere With Natural Elements

Incorporating natural elements into your home is a powerful way to reduce environmental stressors and create a calming atmosphere. Natural elements like plants, wood, and stone help ground us, providing a sense of tranquility and connection to nature. Additionally, natural materials are often less toxic than synthetic ones, promoting a healthier indoor environment.

Incorporating Natural Elements for a Balanced Environment

- **Add Indoor Plants**: Indoor plants add color, improve air quality, and bring a touch of nature indoors, creating a calming effect and reducing stress.

- **Use Natural Materials**: Choose materials like wood, bamboo, stone, or wool for furniture, flooring, and decor to create a warm, grounded atmosphere.

- **Include Water Elements**: Small indoor water features, like fountains or tabletop waterfalls, add soothing sounds and promote relaxation.

- **Decorate with Natural Colors**: Soft, earthy tones create a serene environment. Colors like green, beige, and light blue evoke natural landscapes, enhancing the calming atmosphere.

Incorporating natural elements in your home brings the benefits of the outdoors inside, fostering a balanced and restorative living space.

Conclusion: Embracing a Low-Stress, Health-Focused Environment

Reducing environmental stressors is an essential part of creating a home that nurtures health, well-being, and sustainability. By addressing factors like noise, air quality, lighting, and EMFs, and by incorporating natural elements and mindful design, you can transform your space into a sanctuary that supports relaxation, focus, and physical health.

As you integrate these practices into your daily life, remember that each small change contributes to a more balanced, health-promoting environment. By consciously reducing environmental stressors, you enhance not only your personal well-being but also your connection to the world around you. Embrace this journey to create a home that aligns with your values, protects your health, and provides a peaceful retreat from the demands of the outside world.

CHAPTER 9: SUSTAINABLE MINDSET: THE MENTAL HEALTH BENEFITS OF GREEN LIVING

Green living isn't just about recycling, conserving energy, or reducing waste—it's a way of life that can transform our mental health and emotional well-being. A sustainable mindset allows us to reconnect with nature, cultivate mindfulness, and find purpose in our daily choices. This chapter will explore the many ways that a green lifestyle positively impacts mental health, providing actionable steps to build a sustainable mindset that nurtures both the planet and our inner lives.

From reducing eco-anxiety to practicing gratitude, we'll delve into how living sustainably fosters peace, reduces stress, and enhances a sense of meaning. By aligning our actions with eco-friendly values, we can live a balanced life that benefits our mental health and the environment.

1. The Link Between Sustainability And Mental Health

In recent years, researchers have found strong connections between sustainable living and mental well-being. Environmental challenges like climate change, pollution, and resource depletion can lead to feelings of overwhelm, stress, and even eco-anxiety. A sustainable lifestyle, however, empowers individuals to take positive action, creating a sense of agency and purpose. This mindset shift not only helps protect the environment but also promotes emotional resilience, reducing anxiety and improving mood.

Mental Health Benefits of a Sustainable Lifestyle

- **Reduced Anxiety**: By taking concrete actions to care for the planet, people often feel a greater sense of control, which reduces feelings of eco-anxiety and helplessness.

- **Increased Sense of Purpose**: Living sustainably aligns actions with personal values, fostering a deep sense of purpose and fulfillment.

- **Mindfulness and Presence**: Sustainable practices encourage mindfulness, helping individuals become more aware of their surroundings and live in the present moment.

- **Boosted Self-Esteem**: Making eco-friendly choices that benefit the community and the planet can lead to higher self-esteem and feelings of accomplishment.

Understanding the mental health benefits of green living offers a compelling reason to embrace sustainability as a way of nurturing both ourselves and the world.

2. Cultivating Eco-Mindfulness: Living In Harmony With Nature

Mindfulness is the practice of being fully present and engaged with the current moment. Eco-mindfulness extends this awareness to our relationship with the environment, encouraging us to notice and appreciate the natural world around us. This practice not only fosters a sense of connection with nature but also reduces stress and promotes mental clarity.

Practical Ways to Practice Eco-Mindfulness

1. **Mindful Nature Walks**: Take slow, intentional walks in natural settings, observing the colors, sounds, and scents around you. Allow yourself to be fully present, noticing each detail without judgment.

2. **Savoring Eco-Friendly Routines**: Perform everyday tasks, like preparing a plant-based meal or tending to a garden, with full awareness, appreciating the sensory aspects of each step.

3. **Gratitude for Natural Resources**: Practice gratitude by acknowledging the natural resources that support your life, from clean air and water to the food on your plate.

4. **Create a Nature Connection Ritual**: Set aside time each day to connect with nature, whether it's sitting outside, watching the sunrise, or watering houseplants.

Eco-mindfulness fosters an appreciation for the natural world, creating a sense of calm and purpose that enhances overall mental well-being.

3. Reducing Eco-Anxiety: Taking Action For Peace Of Mind

Eco-anxiety, or the fear and concern over environmental decline, is an increasingly common experience. While awareness of environmental issues is essential, the constant barrage of alarming news can lead to feelings of helplessness, sadness, and stress. Adopting a sustainable mindset helps combat eco-anxiety by empowering individuals to take meaningful action, fostering hope and resilience.

Strategies for Managing Eco-Anxiety

- **Focus on Small, Positive Actions**: Recognize that every small step counts, whether it's reducing plastic use, conserving energy, or buying secondhand. Small, consistent actions build a sense of progress and hope.

- **Join a Community or Group**: Being part of an environmental group or community not only magnifies your impact but also provides support, encouragement, and a sense of belonging.

- **Limit Media Exposure**: While staying informed is important, excessive exposure to environmental news can lead to overwhelm. Set boundaries for media consumption, and focus on positive news whenever possible.

- **Practice Self-Compassion**: Remember that nobody can be "perfectly" sustainable. Practicing eco-friendly habits is about progress, not perfection. Celebrate your efforts without guilt or self-criticism.

By focusing on manageable, positive actions, you can reduce eco-anxiety, build resilience, and maintain hope in the face of environmental challenges.

4. Embracing Minimalism For A Clear Mind And Balanced Life

Minimalism is an approach to living that values quality over quantity, encouraging us to own less and appreciate more. A minimalist lifestyle reduces environmental impact by curbing excessive consumption and waste, while also creating mental clarity, reducing stress, and enhancing focus. By removing clutter—both physical and mental—minimalism cultivates a sense of calm and intentionality.

Benefits of Minimalism for Mental Health

- **Reduced Stress**: Simplifying your surroundings decreases visual clutter, which can reduce mental stress and create a sense of peace.

- **Increased Focus**: A minimalist environment limits distractions, enhancing focus and mental clarity.

- **Sense of Freedom**: Letting go of unnecessary possessions promotes a sense of freedom and lightness, allowing more time and energy for meaningful pursuits.

- **Enhanced Gratitude**: By valuing quality over quantity, minimalism fosters gratitude for the things you do own, encouraging appreciation and contentment.

Practical Steps to Embrace Minimalism

1. **Start Small**: Begin by decluttering one room, drawer, or shelf at a time, assessing what truly adds value to your life.

2. **Adopt the "One In, One Out" Rule**: For every new item you bring into your home, let go of one that no longer serves a purpose. This helps prevent clutter accumulation.

3. **Focus on Experiences Over Things**: Prioritize

meaningful experiences, such as spending time in nature or learning new skills, over purchasing material goods.

4. **Regularly Reevaluate Your Belongings**: Minimalism is an ongoing process. Periodically revisit your possessions and consider donating, recycling, or repurposing items that no longer serve you.

Embracing minimalism allows you to create a balanced, eco-friendly space that promotes calm, mental clarity, and intentional living.

5. Building A Sense Of Purpose Through Sustainable Habits

Purpose is a fundamental element of well-being. Living sustainably aligns our actions with values, creating a sense of purpose that enhances life satisfaction and mental resilience. When we feel that our choices are meaningful and positively impact the world, we experience a sense of fulfillment and motivation.

Ways to Cultivate Purpose through Green Living

- **Set Sustainable Goals**: Define personal sustainability goals, such as reducing plastic waste, conserving water, or switching to a plant-based diet. Working toward these goals fosters a sense of achievement and purpose.

- **Volunteer for Environmental Causes**: Volunteering with environmental organizations, community clean-ups, or conservation efforts connects you to a larger purpose, providing social connections and a sense of fulfillment.

- **Educate and Inspire Others**: Sharing your sustainable journey with family, friends, or through social media can inspire others and deepen your own commitment to green living.

- **Track Your Impact**: Tracking your environmental impact—such as carbon footprint reduction or waste saved—provides a tangible reminder of the positive changes you're making, reinforcing a sense of purpose.

Sustainable habits contribute to a life filled with meaning, offering mental and emotional benefits that enhance well-being.

6. Practicing Gratitude For A Sustainable Life

Gratitude is a powerful practice that fosters positivity, reduces stress, and improves mental health. In the context of green living, gratitude helps us appreciate the natural resources and beauty around us, cultivating a mindset of abundance and respect for the environment. By practicing gratitude regularly, we shift from a mindset of consumption to one of appreciation, promoting sustainability and well-being.

Simple Gratitude Practices for Sustainable Living

- **Daily Gratitude Journal**: Write down three things each day that you're grateful for—whether it's a beautiful sunset, a meaningful conversation, or the fresh air you breathe.

- **Express Appreciation for Nature**: Acknowledge the beauty of nature whenever possible. Take a moment to appreciate the trees, the weather, or even the houseplants in your home.

- **Mindful Consumption**: When you make purchases, practice gratitude by recognizing the resources, labor, and energy that brought the item to you.

- **Give Back to the Planet**: Show gratitude for the Earth by engaging in eco-friendly acts, like planting trees, supporting local farmers, or cleaning up a park.

Gratitude helps us develop a respectful and mindful relationship with the environment, leading to a life of fulfillment and balanced mental health.

7. Cultivating Resilience Through Sustainable Living

Sustainable living encourages resilience, teaching us to adapt, be resourceful, and find creative solutions to challenges. By practicing sustainability, we develop the flexibility to handle difficult situations and the emotional strength to face environmental challenges with hope and determination.

Ways to Build Resilience through Green Living

- **Embrace Imperfection**: Understand that sustainable living is a journey, and it's okay not to be perfect. Allow yourself to make mistakes, learn, and grow.

- **Adapt to New Habits Gradually**: Introduce sustainable habits gradually rather than all at once. Adjusting slowly builds resilience and increases the likelihood of long-term success.

- **Find Inspiration in Nature's Resilience**: Observe how nature adapts and regenerates, even in difficult conditions. Let nature's resilience serve as inspiration for your own journey.

- **Reflect on Progress**: Regularly take stock of how far you've come in your sustainable journey. Recognizing progress builds confidence and resilience, reinforcing your commitment to green living.

Sustainable living not only fosters mental resilience but also instills a sense of adaptability that can benefit all aspects of life.

Conclusion: Embracing a Sustainable Mindset for Holistic Well-Being

A sustainable mindset goes beyond eco-friendly actions—it's a way of living that brings purpose, peace, and positivity into every aspect of life. By aligning our daily choices with environmental values, we create a life of meaning, reduced stress, and connection to the natural world. Sustainable living promotes mental well-being by reducing anxiety, fostering gratitude, encouraging mindfulness, and nurturing resilience.

As you continue your journey, remember that sustainability is not about perfection, but about intentionality and growth. Each small step you take toward a sustainable mindset brings you closer to a life that's fulfilling, balanced, and deeply connected to the planet. Embrace green living as a pathway to holistic well-being, a lifestyle that honors both the Earth and your inner peace.

CHAPTER 10: CULTIVATING COMMUNITY AND CONNECTION

Living sustainably doesn't have to be a solitary journey. In fact, community is a fundamental part of the sustainable lifestyle, bringing people together with a shared purpose and creating a network of support and inspiration. By joining others in environmental initiatives and learning together, we can strengthen our commitment to sustainability, expand our impact, and find fulfillment through connection and collaboration.

In this chapter, we'll explore the many ways that community and connection contribute to a more sustainable lifestyle and greater well-being. From volunteering and attending local events to starting your own sustainability group, this chapter will guide you through building a supportive, eco-conscious community that fosters purpose, resilience, and joy.

1. The Power Of Community In Sustainable Living

Community offers a powerful way to amplify sustainable practices, creating collective change that's greater than any one person could achieve alone. The relationships we build through shared goals and interests provide encouragement, motivation, and accountability on our sustainability journey. In a supportive community, sustainable living becomes easier, more enjoyable, and more impactful.

Benefits of Community for Sustainable Living

- **Shared Knowledge and Resources**: Being part of a community allows individuals to share resources, ideas, and practical solutions for living sustainably.

- **Increased Motivation and Accountability**: Knowing that others are working alongside you toward the same goals can strengthen your commitment to green habits.

- **Emotional Support**: Community provides emotional support for those facing eco-anxiety, burnout, or challenges related to sustainable living.

- **Collective Impact**: When people work together, they can achieve larger, community-wide sustainability goals, such as waste reduction or environmental conservation.

Understanding the role of community in sustainable living highlights the importance of connection as a pathway to a meaningful, balanced life.

2. Finding Like-Minded Individuals For Support And Inspiration

Connecting with like-minded individuals offers valuable support and inspiration on your journey toward sustainable living. Whether it's through local events, online groups, or volunteer opportunities, surrounding yourself with people who share your values provides encouragement, new perspectives, and friendship.

Ways to Find Like-Minded Individuals

1. **Attend Local Sustainability Events**: Check local listings for events such as eco-markets, workshops, and talks on sustainability topics. These gatherings are a great way to meet people who share your interests.

2. **Join Environmental Groups**: Many communities have organizations focused on conservation, gardening, wildlife protection, or recycling. Joining a group like this can introduce you to people who are passionate about making a positive impact.

3. **Participate in Online Communities**: Digital platforms offer countless online groups and forums where people discuss sustainability topics. Look for Facebook groups, subreddits, or apps dedicated to green living, where you can exchange ideas and find support.

4. **Attend Classes and Workshops**: Participate in sustainability classes or workshops, such as composting, urban gardening, or eco-friendly DIY crafts. These spaces are not only educational but also create opportunities for connection.

Finding your community provides encouragement and accountability, making sustainable living more fulfilling and enjoyable.

3. Creating Your Own Sustainability Group Or Initiative

If you're passionate about sustainability and have a vision for bringing people together, consider creating your own sustainability group or initiative. Starting a group allows you to shape its mission, build a support network, and drive positive change within your community.

Steps to Start a Sustainability Group

- **Define Your Mission and Goals**: Decide what you want the group to achieve, such as reducing waste, promoting local farming, or organizing community clean-ups. Clearly defined goals provide direction and purpose for the group.

- **Gather Initial Members**: Start by inviting friends, family, or neighbors who might be interested. Social media and community boards are also great ways to attract new members.

- **Plan Activities and Events**: Schedule regular meetings and organize activities like litter clean-ups, sustainable living workshops, or community garden projects to engage members and make a tangible impact.

- **Partner with Local Organizations**: Collaborate with local businesses, schools, or environmental organizations to expand your group's reach and access resources.

- **Celebrate Progress and Milestones**: Recognize the group's achievements, both big and small. Celebrating progress reinforces commitment and keeps members motivated.

Starting your own initiative can bring a sense of purpose and empowerment as you see the positive impact your group creates.

4. Participating In Community Gardening And Urban Agriculture

Community gardens and urban agriculture projects are popular, effective ways to promote sustainability, reduce food waste, and build community. Gardening with others creates shared responsibility and provides a tangible way to connect with the environment, grow healthy food, and support local ecosystems.

Benefits of Community Gardening

- **Promotes Food Security**: Community gardens provide fresh, affordable produce, promoting food security and reducing dependency on food transportation.

- **Builds Community Connections**: Gardening together fosters collaboration, creating a strong sense of camaraderie among participants.

- **Reduces Environmental Impact**: Growing food locally reduces the carbon footprint associated with transportation, packaging, and waste.

- **Improves Mental Health**: Working with plants and soil has been shown to reduce stress, increase happiness, and provide a sense of accomplishment.

Getting Involved in Community Gardens

1. **Find Local Gardens**: Many cities have community gardens where residents can rent plots or volunteer to help with shared gardening spaces.

2. **Start a Garden in Your Neighborhood**: If no community garden exists nearby, consider starting one. Work with local authorities, secure a plot of land, and recruit neighbors who are interested.

3. **Join a Garden Co-Op**: Some communities have garden co-ops, where participants share the work and the produce, reducing individual responsibilities and

costs.

4. **Attend Workshops and Events**: Many community gardens host events like harvest festivals, gardening workshops, and cooking demonstrations, which are great for learning and connecting.

Community gardening supports sustainable food practices while fostering connection and personal well-being.

5. Volunteering For Environmental Causes

Volunteering is a fulfilling way to support sustainability efforts, meet like-minded people, and give back to the community. Volunteering allows you to contribute to environmental protection while learning new skills, building friendships, and gaining a sense of accomplishment.

Types of Environmental Volunteer Opportunities

- **Wildlife Conservation Projects**: Volunteer with organizations that protect endangered species, conserve habitats, or rehabilitate injured wildlife.

- **Tree Planting Initiatives**: Join reforestation projects, which help restore natural ecosystems, absorb CO_2, and prevent soil erosion.

- **Beach and Park Clean-Ups**: Participate in clean-up events, where volunteers remove litter from natural areas, protecting wildlife and reducing pollution.

- **Environmental Education**: Volunteer with educational programs that teach communities about sustainability, conservation, and green practices.

Tips for Finding Volunteer Opportunities

1. **Check Local Organizations**: Many environmental groups, such as the Sierra Club or the World Wildlife Fund, organize local volunteer events.

2. **Visit Volunteer Websites**: Websites like VolunteerMatch, Idealist, and local environmental sites list volunteer opportunities for various causes and skill levels.

3. **Ask at Community Centers**: Local community centers or libraries often host or support volunteer events, providing information on ways to get involved.

4. **Bring Friends or Family Along**: Volunteering with

others can make the experience more enjoyable and strengthen bonds with loved ones who share your values.

Volunteering not only enhances community connection but also provides personal fulfillment and hands-on experience in sustainable practices.

6. Supporting Local And Sustainable Businesses

Supporting local and sustainable businesses is a powerful way to promote eco-friendly practices while strengthening the community's economy. Local businesses often have a smaller environmental footprint than large corporations, and many focus on sustainable practices such as sourcing locally, minimizing waste, and prioritizing fair labor.

Ways to Support Sustainable Businesses

- **Shop Locally**: Prioritize shopping at local farmers' markets, independent stores, and eco-conscious businesses, which often have a lower carbon footprint.

- **Research Brands**: Look for businesses that are committed to sustainable practices, such as using recycled materials, offering eco-friendly products, or supporting local suppliers.

- **Choose B Corporations**: B Corporations are companies certified for meeting high environmental and social standards. Supporting B Corps ensures your money goes to businesses with responsible practices.

- **Share Your Experiences**: Write positive reviews, recommend sustainable brands to friends, and share your experiences on social media to encourage others to support eco-conscious businesses.

By choosing sustainable businesses, you contribute to a thriving local economy and a healthier environment, while supporting companies that align with your values.

7. Organizing And Participating In Community Sustainability Events

Community events focused on sustainability offer opportunities to learn, connect, and take action with others. These events provide a platform for sharing knowledge, raising awareness, and inspiring collective change. Organizing or attending local events amplifies the message of sustainability and strengthens community bonds.

Types of Community Sustainability Events

- **Eco-Fairs and Markets**: These events bring together vendors, artisans, and organizations focused on eco-friendly products, sustainable practices, and local goods.

- **Educational Workshops**: Host or attend workshops on topics like composting, sustainable gardening, or DIY green projects.

- **Swap and Share Events**: Organize events where people can swap items like clothing, books, or household goods, promoting reuse and reducing waste.

- **Film Screenings and Discussions**: Show documentaries on environmental topics followed by group discussions, inspiring thoughtful dialogue and action.

Tips for Organizing a Community Event

1. **Choose a Theme**: Pick a theme that resonates with your community's needs and interests, such as zero-waste living, local farming, or climate action.

2. **Collaborate with Local Partners**: Reach out to local businesses, schools, and environmental organizations for support, resources, and promotion.

3. **Promote the Event**: Use social media, community

boards, and word of mouth to promote the event and encourage participation.

4. **Make It Fun and Inclusive**: Create an inviting atmosphere with activities for all ages, food options, and interactive workshops.

Community events provide an engaging way for people to learn about sustainability and form connections that support ongoing change.

8. Building A Sense Of Collective Responsibility And Purpose

A key aspect of cultivating community and connection in sustainability is fostering a sense of collective responsibility and purpose. By working together, communities can make a greater impact, inspire others, and build resilience. This shared sense of responsibility motivates individuals to stay committed to their green practices, knowing they are part of something larger.

Ways to Foster Collective Responsibility

- **Establish Shared Goals**: Define common goals, such as waste reduction or energy conservation, that everyone in the community can work toward.

- **Celebrate Group Successes**: Acknowledge and celebrate milestones, like reaching recycling goals or planting trees, to reinforce a sense of collective achievement.

- **Encourage Youth Involvement**: Engage young people in sustainability efforts, as they bring fresh ideas and energy, fostering a culture of environmental stewardship for future generations.

- **Share Stories of Impact**: Highlight stories of individuals or groups making a difference, showing how small actions contribute to collective change.

By nurturing a shared sense of purpose, you build a resilient community that is dedicated to creating a sustainable future.

Conclusion: Embracing Connection for a Sustainable Future

Cultivating community and connection is a cornerstone of sustainable living, providing support, motivation, and a sense of belonging on our green journey. By joining hands with others, sharing knowledge, and working toward common goals, we can create a meaningful, positive impact that benefits both our communities and the planet.

Embrace the power of community as you pursue a sustainable lifestyle. Together, we can foster a world where eco-friendly practices are the norm, support one another in times of change, and find joy and purpose in the pursuit of a more sustainable future. Through community, sustainable living becomes more than an individual journey—it becomes a shared mission, creating lasting bonds, collective purpose, and a brighter world for all.

CHAPTER 11: THE NEXT STEPS: BUILDING SUSTAINABLE HABITS FOR LIFE

Living sustainably is a journey that often begins with small, intentional changes. However, the challenge lies in maintaining these practices over the long term, especially in a world that constantly promotes convenience and consumption. The key to lasting change is habit formation—turning sustainable actions into automatic, ingrained behaviors that become part of everyday life.

In this chapter, we'll explore the science behind habit formation, practical strategies for developing and sustaining eco-friendly habits, and methods for adapting and evolving these habits over time. By focusing on building habits, you'll create a lifestyle that supports both personal well-being and the planet, ultimately leading to a fulfilling, purpose-driven life.

1. Understanding The Psychology Of Habit Formation

Before diving into practical strategies, it's helpful to understand the psychology of habit formation. Habits are behaviors that have become automatic through repetition and reinforcement. Forming a habit involves creating a loop consisting of three parts: a cue, a routine, and a reward. This loop helps us adopt new behaviors and repeat them consistently until they become second nature.

The Habit Loop

- **Cue**: A cue is a trigger that initiates the habit. For example, seeing a reusable water bottle on your desk can remind you to drink water instead of reaching for a disposable plastic bottle.

- **Routine**: The routine is the action itself, such as filling up the reusable bottle with water. Consistently performing the action builds the habit.

- **Reward**: The reward reinforces the behavior, making it more likely you'll repeat it. In this case, staying hydrated and reducing plastic waste provides a feeling of satisfaction and accomplishment.

By understanding how habits work, you can intentionally create cues, routines, and rewards that support your sustainable goals.

2. Starting Small: The Power Of Tiny Habits

One of the most effective strategies for building lasting habits is to start small. Research shows that small changes are more manageable, less overwhelming, and easier to sustain over time. By focusing on tiny habits, you create momentum and build confidence, making it easier to progress toward larger sustainable goals.

Examples of Tiny Sustainable Habits

1. **Carry a Reusable Bag**: Start by bringing one reusable bag with you when you go shopping, reducing the need for plastic bags.

2. **Turn Off Lights**: Get into the habit of turning off lights when leaving a room to conserve energy.

3. **Use a Reusable Coffee Cup**: Start by bringing your own coffee cup just once a week, then gradually increase frequency as it becomes a habit.

4. **Shorten Showers by One Minute**: Reducing shower time by a single minute conserves water, and this habit can be built on over time.

Focusing on these small changes allows you to experience success without becoming overwhelmed, creating a foundation for more substantial habits.

3. Setting Clear And Achievable Goals

Clear, achievable goals make it easier to stay motivated and measure your progress. When setting goals, try to make them specific, realistic, and time-bound, as this increases the likelihood of success. For example, instead of aiming to "reduce waste," you could set a goal to "bring reusable containers to the grocery store every Saturday for the next month."

Tips for Setting Sustainable Goals

- **Be Specific**: Clearly define what you want to achieve, such as "reduce plastic waste by using glass containers for leftovers."

- **Set a Timeline**: Give yourself a timeframe to accomplish the goal, such as "use a reusable water bottle every day for the next month."

- **Track Progress**: Keep a record of your achievements, which serves as a reminder of how far you've come and reinforces your commitment.

- **Celebrate Milestones**: Acknowledge and celebrate small wins, like completing a week or month of your new habit, to maintain motivation.

Goal-setting creates a structured pathway to sustainable habits, giving you a sense of purpose and direction.

4. Creating A Sustainable Environment To Support Habits

Your environment plays a significant role in shaping behavior. By making small adjustments to your surroundings, you can encourage eco-friendly actions and reduce the likelihood of unsustainable choices. A well-designed environment acts as a constant reminder of your commitment to sustainability.

Tips for Designing a Habit-Supportive Environment

- **Place Reusable Items in Visible Spots**: Keep reusable bags, containers, and water bottles in convenient, visible locations to remind yourself to use them.

- **Organize Recycling and Composting Areas**: Create a designated space for recycling and composting that's easily accessible, making it more likely you'll stick to these habits.

- **Remove Single-Use Items**: Replace single-use items with sustainable alternatives in the kitchen, bathroom, and workspaces to reduce waste automatically.

- **Add Reminders and Visual Cues**: Use sticky notes or eco-friendly labels to remind yourself of sustainable actions, like reducing energy use or conserving water.

An environment that supports sustainable habits reduces resistance and makes it easier to stay on track.

5. Building Accountability For Long-Term Success

Accountability is a powerful motivator for maintaining habits, especially when forming new, eco-friendly behaviors. Sharing your goals with others, joining sustainability groups, or partnering with friends can reinforce your commitment and provide support.

Ways to Build Accountability

- **Share Your Goals with Friends or Family**: Telling others about your goals creates a sense of responsibility, as you'll be more motivated to stick to your habits.

- **Join a Sustainability Group**: Being part of an eco-conscious community provides encouragement, support, and accountability as you work toward your goals.

- **Use Habit-Tracking Apps**: Many apps allow you to track habits, set reminders, and see your progress over time, creating accountability and visual reinforcement.

- **Partner with a "Sustainability Buddy"**: Find a friend who shares similar goals and check in regularly to support each other's progress.

Accountability helps you stay motivated, making it more likely that sustainable habits become an enduring part of your lifestyle.

6. Overcoming Challenges And Building Resilience

Like any lifestyle change, building sustainable habits comes with challenges. From busy schedules to occasional setbacks, life can sometimes disrupt even the best intentions. Developing resilience and learning to overcome obstacles is essential for maintaining a sustainable lifestyle over time.

Strategies for Overcoming Challenges

- **Anticipate Obstacles**: Think ahead about possible barriers, like time constraints or lack of resources, and plan solutions, such as prepping reusable bags in advance.

- **Practice Self-Compassion**: Be kind to yourself when you face setbacks. Sustainable living is a journey, and it's natural to experience challenges along the way.

- **Reframe Setbacks as Learning Opportunities**: Instead of seeing challenges as failures, view them as opportunities to learn and adapt. Ask yourself what you can do differently next time.

- **Revisit and Adjust Goals**: If a habit isn't working, adjust it to better fit your lifestyle. Flexibility allows you to adapt to changes while staying committed to sustainability.

Resilience helps you adapt and find creative solutions, making it easier to continue building and maintaining sustainable habits.

7. Keeping Motivation Alive With Purpose And Reflection

Motivation is essential for sustaining habits, and one of the best ways to stay motivated is to connect with the deeper purpose behind your sustainable choices. Reflecting on the impact of your actions, celebrating progress, and reminding yourself of your goals can reignite your motivation over time.

Ways to Maintain Motivation

- **Reflect on Your "Why"**: Regularly remind yourself of why you're committed to sustainability, whether it's for environmental health, personal well-being, or future generations.

- **Track Your Impact**: Keep a record of your progress, such as the amount of plastic saved, waste reduced, or energy conserved. Seeing your impact in tangible terms reinforces motivation.

- **Reward Yourself**: Celebrate milestones by treating yourself to experiences or rewards that align with your values, such as a nature walk or a sustainably-made item.

- **Find Inspiration in Nature**: Spend time outdoors, observing the beauty and resilience of nature. This connection often rekindles the desire to protect and preserve the environment.

Reflecting on the purpose behind your habits keeps you grounded and motivated, making sustainable living more meaningful and enjoyable.

8. Adapting And Evolving Sustainable Habits Over Time

Sustainable living is a dynamic journey, and habits may need to evolve over time to reflect new insights, changes in lifestyle, or advances in eco-friendly practices. By remaining flexible and open to adaptation, you'll be able to refine your habits and continue progressing on your sustainable path.

Tips for Evolving Your Sustainable Habits

- **Reevaluate Your Goals Regularly**: Periodically revisit your sustainable goals to ensure they align with your current values, interests, and lifestyle.

- **Embrace New Sustainable Practices**: Stay informed about new technologies, ideas, and practices in sustainability, and consider integrating them into your routine.

- **Experiment with Alternative Habits**: Test new ways of approaching old habits. For example, if you've mastered using reusable bags, consider experimenting with zero-waste grocery shopping.

- **Seek Continuous Learning**: Attend workshops, read books, or join discussions to deepen your understanding of sustainability and learn how to incorporate new habits.

Adapting habits over time helps you maintain momentum, allowing sustainable living to become a natural and enjoyable part of your life.

9. Building A Legacy Of Sustainable Living

Sustainable habits don't just impact your life—they create a legacy for future generations. By modeling eco-friendly behaviors and sharing your journey, you inspire others to adopt similar habits, creating a ripple effect that extends far beyond your immediate actions. This legacy of sustainability is a powerful motivator, as it reminds us that each small action contributes to a brighter, more sustainable future.

Ways to Build a Legacy of Sustainable Living

- **Involve Family and Friends**: Share your sustainable practices with loved ones, teaching them how to incorporate eco-friendly habits into their lives.

- **Educate and Inspire Others**: Whether through social media, blog posts, or casual conversations, sharing your journey can inspire others to adopt sustainable practices.

- **Mentor Younger Generations**: Pass on sustainable habits to younger family members, teaching them the importance of protecting the environment.

- **Support Community Initiatives**: Contribute to local sustainability projects or community efforts, creating a collective legacy that benefits the wider community.

Building a legacy of sustainable living fosters a sense of purpose and connection, reinforcing the impact of your choices and inspiring others to continue the journey.

Conclusion: Embracing Sustainable Habits for a Lifetime

Building sustainable habits is more than a lifestyle choice; it's a lifelong journey toward meaningful, intentional living. By starting small, setting achievable goals, creating supportive environments, and staying motivated, you'll cultivate habits that support both personal well-being and planetary health. These habits are the foundation of a life that aligns with your values, bringing fulfillment, resilience, and a deep sense of purpose.

Embrace this journey of sustainable habit formation, knowing that each action—no matter how small—contributes to a healthier, more balanced life and a brighter, greener world. Through perseverance, reflection, and adaptability, you can transform sustainability from a goal into a way of life, creating a legacy that inspires future generations to live in harmony with the Earth.

CHAPTER 12: LIVING GREEN FOR FUTURE GENERATIONS

Sustainable living is about more than making eco-friendly choices for ourselves—it's about building a better world for those who come after us. Every action we take has a ripple effect, influencing not only our immediate surroundings but also the legacy we leave for future generations. Living green for future generations means embracing sustainable practices, modeling environmental stewardship, and fostering values that encourage respect for the planet.

In this chapter, we'll explore ways to create a lasting impact through sustainable choices, with a focus on educating, inspiring, and empowering the next generation. By instilling eco-friendly values, sharing knowledge, and fostering a connection to nature, we can help ensure that the progress we make today extends far into the future.

1. Understanding The Concept Of Environmental Legacy

An environmental legacy refers to the lasting impact of our actions on the planet and future generations. This legacy includes the choices we make about resource use, waste management, and environmental stewardship. Leaving a positive environmental legacy requires intentionality, focusing on practices that protect and sustain the Earth.

The Importance of an Environmental Legacy

- **Protecting Natural Resources**: Preserving clean air, water, and soil ensures that future generations can meet their basic needs.

- **Fostering Resilience**: Sustainable practices increase resilience against climate change, resource shortages, and other environmental challenges.

- **Promoting Long-Term Health**: Reducing pollution, chemical exposure, and waste improves the health and well-being of both current and future generations.

- **Creating a Culture of Environmental Stewardship**: By living sustainably, we model values and behaviors that inspire others to adopt eco-friendly practices, creating a culture that prioritizes environmental health.

Understanding our environmental legacy encourages us to make choices that benefit not only ourselves but also those who will inherit the Earth.

2. Fostering Environmental Stewardship At Home

Our homes are the first places where we can begin to build an environmental legacy. By creating a home environment that models sustainable living, we lay a foundation for future generations to carry forward. This includes practicing eco-friendly habits, minimizing waste, and teaching family members about the importance of protecting the planet.

Ways to Foster Environmental Stewardship at Home

1. **Practice Conscious Consumption**: Choose durable, eco-friendly products, avoid unnecessary purchases, and opt for quality over quantity to reduce waste.

2. **Model Sustainable Habits**: Show family members, especially children, how to reduce waste, recycle properly, and conserve resources through your actions.

3. **Prioritize Non-Toxic Living**: Use non-toxic cleaning products, choose natural furnishings, and limit plastic use to create a healthier home for all occupants.

4. **Incorporate Nature into Your Space**: Add houseplants, create an outdoor garden, or set up a bird feeder to bring nature closer, fostering appreciation for the environment.

By fostering environmental stewardship at home, you create a space that values sustainability and respects the natural world.

3. Teaching Sustainability To Younger Generations

Educating young people about sustainability is essential for building a lasting environmental legacy. Children and teenagers are more likely to carry forward eco-friendly habits and values if they grow up understanding their importance. Teaching sustainability to younger generations empowers them to make informed choices and become advocates for the planet.

Strategies for Teaching Sustainability

- **Lead by Example**: Children learn by observing, so make eco-friendly practices visible in your daily life. Actions like recycling, composting, and conserving water are lessons in themselves.

- **Encourage Hands-On Learning**: Engage young people in activities that promote environmental awareness, such as gardening, composting, and participating in nature walks.

- **Incorporate Sustainability in Education**: Provide books, documentaries, and resources that explain environmental issues in an age-appropriate way. Many educational materials focus on topics like recycling, conservation, and climate change.

- **Celebrate Eco-Friendly Choices**: Acknowledge and celebrate children's eco-friendly choices, such as picking up litter, choosing reusable items, or helping with recycling tasks.

Teaching sustainability helps young people build a lifelong commitment to protecting the Earth, encouraging a new generation of environmentally conscious individuals.

4. Creating Traditions That Celebrate Nature And Sustainability

Traditions shape family values, build memories, and create a sense of continuity. Establishing family traditions that celebrate nature and sustainability encourages young people to see the environment as something worth protecting. These traditions can become meaningful annual events, creating lifelong memories and a lasting connection to nature.

Eco-Friendly Tradition Ideas

1. **Annual Tree Planting**: Plant a tree together every year, whether on your property, in a local park, or through a reforestation project. This simple act is a symbolic commitment to the environment.

2. **Nature Exploration Days**: Designate a monthly or seasonal day to explore nature, whether hiking in a nearby park, visiting a botanical garden, or camping.

3. **Eco-Friendly Holiday Practices**: For holidays, opt for sustainable decorations, handmade gifts, or activities like crafting with natural materials to reduce waste and celebrate sustainably.

4. **Seasonal Harvesting and Cooking**: Create traditions around seasonal cooking, such as picking apples in the fall, visiting farmers' markets, or planting a vegetable garden. These traditions teach respect for seasonal cycles and the importance of local food.

By establishing nature-focused traditions, you foster a lasting appreciation for the environment and promote eco-friendly values in future generations.

5. Supporting Environmental Education And Advocacy

Supporting environmental education initiatives and advocacy efforts amplifies your impact, contributing to a broader culture of sustainability. Whether by donating, volunteering, or participating in community events, engaging in environmental advocacy strengthens efforts to protect the planet.

Ways to Support Environmental Education and Advocacy

- **Donate to Environmental Organizations**: Contribute to organizations focused on sustainability, conservation, and environmental education, helping fund research, education, and advocacy efforts.

- **Volunteer for Local Initiatives**: Participate in conservation projects, clean-ups, or educational events that raise awareness and promote sustainable practices.

- **Advocate for Green Policies**: Support policies and legislation that protect the environment by attending town hall meetings, signing petitions, or contacting local representatives.

- **Encourage Environmental Literacy**: Share resources, books, and documentaries about sustainability with others, helping spread knowledge and inspire collective action.

Supporting environmental education and advocacy strengthens the impact of individual actions, creating a wider network of people working toward a sustainable future.

6. Practicing "Intergenerational Thinking"

Intergenerational thinking is the practice of considering how our actions today will impact future generations. This perspective encourages us to make choices that are not only sustainable in the present but also beneficial in the long term. By adopting an intergenerational mindset, we prioritize actions that have a lasting, positive impact on the world we leave behind.

Ways to Embrace Intergenerational Thinking

- **Make Long-Term Investments**: Choose high-quality, durable products that reduce waste and serve future generations, such as quality furniture, heirloom seeds, or reusable items.

- **Conserve Natural Resources**: Adopt practices that protect resources like water, soil, and forests, ensuring they remain available for future generations.

- **Reduce Carbon Footprint**: Opt for low-emission transportation, energy conservation, and plant-based diets to minimize climate impacts for future generations.

- **Encourage Legacy Actions**: Involve children and grandchildren in sustainable practices, such as tree planting or composting, that symbolize the commitment to leaving a healthy planet.

Intergenerational thinking reminds us that our sustainable choices have lasting significance, helping us build a legacy of environmental stewardship.

7. Sharing Sustainable Skills And Knowledge

Passing down skills and knowledge related to sustainable living is one of the most powerful ways to build an environmental legacy. Teaching practical skills like gardening, composting, and DIY repairs equips future generations to live resourcefully and sustainably. Sharing these skills also strengthens connections within families and communities, fostering a culture of sustainability.

Skills to Share with Future Generations

- **Gardening and Food Preservation**: Teaching how to grow food, save seeds, and preserve produce fosters self-sufficiency and reduces reliance on industrial food systems.

- **Composting**: Composting skills help reduce food waste, improve soil health, and create a deeper understanding of nature's nutrient cycles.

- **DIY and Upcycling**: Show how to repair, repurpose, and upcycle items to reduce waste and embrace a zero-waste mindset.

- **Energy Conservation Tips**: Teach simple but effective energy-saving practices, like unplugging electronics, using natural lighting, and maintaining appliances for efficiency.

By sharing sustainable skills, you help future generations live resourcefully, reducing waste and fostering a mindset of self-sufficiency and environmental responsibility.

8. Building A Strong Connection To Nature

A strong connection to nature fosters respect, care, and appreciation for the environment. Encouraging time spent outdoors, developing an understanding of natural cycles, and learning about local ecosystems deepen this connection, making future generations more likely to advocate for the Earth.

Ways to Cultivate a Connection to Nature

- **Encourage Outdoor Exploration**: Spend time outdoors regularly, allowing children and family members to explore, play, and learn from the natural world.

- **Teach Nature Observation Skills**: Show how to observe and appreciate local plants, animals, and ecosystems, fostering curiosity and respect for biodiversity.

- **Involve Kids in Conservation Activities**: Involve children in conservation efforts, such as beach clean-ups or wildlife monitoring, to help them understand the importance of protecting natural spaces.

- **Practice Mindful Time in Nature**: Encourage family members to spend time in nature mindfully, noticing the sights, sounds, and smells. This practice promotes a deep sense of connection to the environment.

Building a connection to nature strengthens environmental awareness and instills a lifelong commitment to sustainability.

9. Creating A Legacy Of Hope And Resilience

Sustainable living is not only about reducing impact; it's also about fostering hope and resilience. Showing future generations that positive change is possible, even through small actions, helps them face environmental challenges with optimism and purpose. A legacy of hope inspires resilience, encouraging future generations to continue the work of sustainability with determination.

Ways to Build Hope and Resilience in Future Generations

- **Highlight Success Stories**: Share stories of successful conservation efforts, green innovations, and positive environmental change to inspire optimism.

- **Focus on Small, Meaningful Actions**: Emphasize that every action counts, whether it's recycling, conserving water, or supporting local food systems, to build a sense of empowerment.

- **Encourage Problem-Solving Skills**: Encourage critical thinking and creativity to approach environmental challenges with solutions-based mindsets.

- **Reinforce the Importance of Community**: Show that working together can create meaningful change, fostering a sense of collective responsibility and hope.

By nurturing hope and resilience, we empower future generations to face environmental challenges with courage, optimism, and an unwavering commitment to the planet.

Conclusion: Living Green
for a Lasting Legacy

Living green for future generations is a commitment to a lifestyle that prioritizes both immediate and long-term well-being for people and the planet. Through intentional actions, education, and connection, we build a legacy of sustainability that endures far beyond our lifetimes. The choices we make today—whether planting a tree, teaching sustainable skills, or fostering a love for nature—lay the foundation for a healthier, more resilient world.

As you continue on your journey, remember that each eco-friendly choice, each shared skill, and each mindful act leaves an indelible mark on the world. By living green for future generations, you contribute to a legacy of stewardship, resilience, and hope, empowering others to protect and cherish the planet for years to come. Embrace this mission, knowing that your commitment to sustainability is a gift that will keep giving, inspiring others and preserving the beauty and wonder of the Earth for generations yet to come.

CHAPTER 13: THE PATH FORWARD —SUSTAINING A LIFETIME OF POSITIVE IMPACT

Sustainable living is more than a series of eco-friendly actions; it's a transformative approach to life that connects our values, daily choices, and relationships with a commitment to the planet. As you close this book, remember that this journey isn't about reaching a final destination but about continually growing, adapting, and making a positive impact on the world around you. This closing chapter brings together the themes and insights covered in each chapter, empowering you to take your sustainable journey forward with confidence, purpose, and joy.

Embrace this path with the understanding that each small action builds toward a larger legacy. By committing to sustainable practices, we leave behind not only a healthier planet but also a world that encourages resilience, empathy, and mindfulness. Let this chapter inspire you to turn the insights gained into enduring habits that will sustain you—and the Earth—for years to come.

1. Embracing A Lifetime Of Sustainable Growth

Living sustainably is a journey of growth and evolution. Each small step you take, whether it's choosing reusable products or committing to waste reduction, compounds over time, building a lifestyle rooted in respect for the environment and intentionality. The most meaningful change often begins with small, simple actions that, when repeated and expanded upon, become lifelong habits.

Reinforcing the Foundation of Sustainable Living

- **Consistency Over Complexity**: Often, the simplest habits are the most impactful. Focusing on small, consistent actions, like using less water or conserving energy, provides a stable foundation for sustainable living.

- **Experimentation and Curiosity**: Each individual's sustainable journey is unique. Experiment with different practices, like composting, zero-waste shopping, or urban gardening, to find what resonates with your lifestyle.

- **Continuous Learning and Adaptation**: New technologies, innovations, and ideas constantly emerge within the field of sustainability. Remain open to learning and evolving, adapting your habits as more effective or accessible methods arise.

- **Fostering Resilience Through Growth**: Sustainable living builds resilience—both personal and environmental—allowing you to adapt to challenges, stay committed through setbacks, and find fulfillment in progress over time.

By embracing sustainable growth, you empower yourself to make lasting changes that resonate with your values and contribute positively to the planet.

2. The Power Of Reflection: Celebrating Progress And Learning From Challenges

Reflection is a vital part of sustaining momentum in sustainable living. Taking time to review your progress allows you to appreciate the steps you've taken, recognize the positive impact of your choices, and identify areas for further growth. Reflection also builds resilience by helping you learn from challenges, reframing setbacks as opportunities for growth and adaptation.

Reflective Practices for Sustainable Living

- **Keep a Sustainable Living Journal**: Track your sustainable actions, from the resources you conserve to the waste you reduce, and write about the emotions, challenges, and rewards of living sustainably. This creates a tangible record of your progress, offering inspiration and insights for the future.

- **Celebrate Successes, Big and Small**: Recognize your achievements, whether it's a week of zero-waste living, switching to a plant-based diet, or advocating for green practices at work. Celebrating milestones boosts morale and reinforces commitment.

- **Acknowledge and Learn from Setbacks**: Not every attempt at sustainable living will go as planned. If you encounter a challenge, such as difficulty maintaining a compost system or forgetting reusable bags, consider what you can do differently next time. Reframing challenges as learning opportunities builds resilience.

- **Revisit Goals Regularly**: Periodically assess your goals, celebrating those you've achieved and refining those that may need adjustment. Adjusting goals over time allows you to stay flexible and continuously motivated.

Reflection transforms sustainable living into an evolving journey, allowing you to appreciate your progress, address challenges, and stay rooted in purpose.

3. Fostering A Deep Connection With Nature

A meaningful connection with nature deepens your commitment to sustainability, grounding you in a sense of purpose and wonder. By spending time in natural spaces, observing seasonal changes, or engaging in nature-based activities, you cultivate an appreciation for the beauty and resilience of the environment.

Ways to Cultivate a Connection to Nature

- **Regular Time Outdoors**: Make time for outdoor experiences, whether it's a weekly nature walk, a weekend hike, or simply sitting in a local park. Being in nature reduces stress, increases mindfulness, and reminds us of the environment we aim to protect.

- **Nature Journaling**: Observe and record details about the natural world around you, such as weather changes, wildlife, or plant growth. Nature journaling fosters a sense of presence and gratitude for the Earth's complexity and beauty.

- **Mindfulness Practices in Nature**: Engage in mindfulness or meditation outdoors, taking time to focus on sounds, smells, and textures around you. Nature-based mindfulness can deepen your appreciation for biodiversity and environmental cycles.

- **Learn About Local Ecosystems**: Understanding the flora, fauna, and natural cycles in your area helps build a sense of responsibility for preserving local ecosystems and habitats.

A deep connection to nature enriches your sustainable journey, encouraging empathy, reverence, and a commitment to environmental stewardship.

4. Strengthening Community And Collective Action For Lasting Impact

While individual actions are powerful, collective efforts amplify impact. Community is essential to sustainable living, providing support, accountability, and shared goals. Working together, we can create a more sustainable society, drive systemic change, and inspire future generations to protect the Earth.

Engaging in Collective Sustainable Action

- **Support Local Environmental Organizations**: Engage with or support groups working on conservation, waste reduction, renewable energy, or biodiversity protection. These organizations strengthen community impact and provide resources to further eco-friendly initiatives.

- **Participate in Local Eco-Initiatives**: Attend community clean-ups, tree-planting events, or zero-waste workshops to connect with others who share your values. Collaborative action magnifies each person's contribution, creating a significant positive impact.

- **Advocate for Sustainable Policies**: Work with others to support policies promoting green energy, biodiversity protection, or plastic reduction. Advocating for these changes within your community adds a powerful voice to the call for systemic change.

- **Educate and Inspire**: Share your sustainable journey with friends, family, and colleagues. Hosting a workshop, leading a book club focused on environmental topics, or simply engaging in open discussions helps inspire others to make sustainable choices.

Building community and participating in collective action

reinforce the importance of sustainable living, ensuring a greater impact and inspiring others to join the movement.

5. Leaving A Legacy Of Environmental Stewardship

A sustainable lifestyle creates a legacy for future generations, ensuring that the Earth's resources are preserved and protected. By teaching others, particularly younger generations, to adopt sustainable practices, we plant seeds for a brighter, more resilient future. Your actions today will echo through the lives of those who come after, fostering a culture of environmental stewardship and respect.

Ways to Build a Sustainable Legacy

- **Mentor and Educate Future Generations**: Pass down sustainable skills such as gardening, composting, and conservation. Teaching young people eco-friendly practices empowers them to make informed, mindful choices.

- **Create Family and Community Traditions**: Establish sustainable family traditions, like annual tree planting, seasonal cooking, or regular nature hikes, to instill a love for nature and conservation.

- **Document Your Sustainable Journey**: Share your progress, successes, and lessons learned with friends, family, or online communities. This documentation serves as a testament to your commitment and as inspiration for others.

- **Lead by Example**: Whether in personal interactions or community efforts, let your sustainable actions speak louder than words. By living your values, you inspire others to join in the journey toward a sustainable future.

Leaving a legacy of stewardship is a gift to future generations, inspiring them to carry forward the work of protecting the planet and its resources.

6. Designing A Life Of Purpose And Fulfillment Through Sustainability

A sustainable lifestyle can provide a sense of purpose that enriches every aspect of life. Living with intention, making mindful choices, and aligning your actions with your values create a fulfilling, purposeful life. This purpose-driven approach to sustainability enhances well-being and brings a sense of peace and joy that extends far beyond material gains.

Creating a Purpose-Driven, Sustainable Life

- **Align Actions with Core Values**: Identify the values that are most important to you, such as conservation, community, or simplicity. Let these values guide your decisions, reinforcing a sense of purpose and alignment.

- **Set Personal and Environmental Goals**: Establish meaningful goals that reflect both personal aspirations and sustainable living. Examples include reducing energy use by a specific percentage, supporting local farms, or transitioning to a plant-based diet.

- **Balance Sustainability with Joy**: Sustainable living doesn't mean sacrifice. Find joy in practices like cooking with seasonal ingredients, creating a beautiful garden, or spending time outdoors, making sustainability a source of fulfillment.

- **Reflect on Your Impact**: Regularly take time to reflect on the positive impact you're making. This reflection reinforces your purpose, reminding you that each small action contributes to a larger vision for a sustainable, balanced life.

A life centered around purpose and sustainability brings deep fulfillment, transforming daily actions into a meaningful legacy.

7. Final Reflections: Living In Harmony With The Earth

Sustainable living is a journey of connection, integrity, and continuous growth. It invites us to harmonize with the Earth, making choices that support the well-being of ourselves, our communities, and the planet. As you embark on this lifelong path, remember that sustainable living isn't about perfection—it's about progress, intention, and the joy of being part of a larger movement.

Principles for a Life in Harmony with the Earth

- **Consistency and Commitment**: Small, consistent actions build a strong foundation for sustainable living. Approach each day with a commitment to do your best, even when challenges arise.

- **Curiosity and Openness**: The world of sustainability is vast and constantly evolving. Stay curious, open to learning, and willing to adapt as new insights emerge.

- **Gratitude for Natural Resources**: Recognize the abundance around you, from clean water to fresh air and nutritious food, fostering a mindset of respect and responsibility.

- **Connection and Empathy**: Sustain a deep connection with nature, recognizing that every choice, no matter how small, impacts the world around us.

Living in harmony with the Earth brings a sense of peace, gratitude, and fulfillment that enriches every area of life.

Conclusion: Embracing Sustainable Living as a Lifelong Journey

As we conclude this journey, remember that sustainable living is a path that extends beyond this book. Each choice, each habit, and each action is part of a larger story—a story of resilience, kindness, and hope. Embrace this journey with intention, knowing that every step forward, no matter how small, makes a difference.

Let this path be filled with purpose, discovery, and joy. Sustainable living is not about reaching a destination; it's about continually striving for a more balanced, compassionate, and eco-friendly way of life. Through each mindful choice, you're building a brighter, more resilient future, leaving a legacy of hope and integrity for generations to come.

By walking this path together, we contribute to a world where sustainable living is the norm—a world that celebrates the Earth's beauty, supports our communities, and empowers future generations to carry forward the work we've begun. Embrace this journey with confidence and joy, knowing that each of us has the power to create positive, lasting change. Together, let's continue to protect, cherish, and sustain the incredible world we call home.

CHAPTER 14: CONCLUSION: A VISION FOR A SUSTAINABLE FUTURE

As we reach the final chapter of this journey, itâ€™s essential to reflect on the impact of each sustainable action and the legacy we collectively create. Sustainable living is not only about the practices we incorporate into our daily lives; itâ€™s about embodying values that contribute to a more balanced, equitable, and healthy world for generations to come. Through this book, we have explored ways to detox our homes, reduce environmental stressors, build community, nurture well-being, and inspire change within our families and social networks. Now, we bring these ideas together, creating a cohesive vision of sustainable living that each of us can carry forward.

In this concluding chapter, weâ€™ll revisit the key themes of the book, reflect on the journey of sustainable living, and look forward to the future with a renewed sense of purpose. By sustaining these efforts over time, we can transform our actions into an enduring commitment to the Earth and all who inhabit it.

1. Revisiting Key Themes: A Holistic Approach To Sustainable Living

Throughout this book, we have seen that sustainable living is more than a series of actions; itâ€™s an approach that permeates every area of life, creating harmony between our personal values and our choices. The journey has been one of self-discovery, intentionality, and resilience, empowering us to become better stewards of our homes, communities, and the planet.

Recap of the Core Principles of Sustainable Living

- **Mindfulness and Awareness**: Sustainable living begins with mindfulness. By being aware of our consumption, waste, and energy use, we gain a clearer understanding of our environmental impact and can make informed decisions that reduce harm to the planet.
- **Health and Wellness Through Eco-Friendly Choices**: Detoxing our homes, choosing non-toxic products, and prioritizing natural materials protect our health while creating safe, vibrant spaces. This approach reflects a commitment to both personal well-being and environmental stewardship.
- **Connection to Community and Nature**: Building connections with like-minded people and embracing a love for nature strengthens our commitment to sustainability, transforming eco-friendly practices into a shared journey.
- **Lifelong Growth and Flexibility**: Sustainable living is a continuous journey of learning and adapting. Flexibility allows us to evolve our habits, respond to new challenges, and make a lasting impact.

These principles serve as guideposts, helping us stay grounded in our values as we move forward in our sustainable journey.

---

2. The Power Of Individual Action: Every Choice Counts

One of the central themes of this book is the power of individual action. Every choice, no matter how small, has a ripple effect, contributing to larger changes within our communities and the environment. By understanding that each decision counts, we empower ourselves to make a meaningful impact, turning everyday actions into a collective force for change.

Examples of Simple Actions with Big Impacts

- **Reducing Plastic Use**: From using reusable bags and water bottles to choosing products with minimal packaging, reducing plastic reduces pollution and conserves resources.
- **Supporting Local and Sustainable Brands**: By choosing to support eco-conscious brands and local businesses, we drive demand for ethical practices and reduce the environmental toll of long-distance shipping.
- **Minimizing Energy Consumption**: Simple acts, like turning off lights, using energy-efficient appliances, or setting up renewable energy options, collectively reduce our carbon footprint.
- **Practicing Conscious Consumption**: Consuming mindfully by buying only what we need, choosing quality over quantity, and reducing waste significantly conserves resources and reduces landfill contributions.

Every sustainable choice builds on the last, adding momentum to a lifestyle that promotes resilience, health, and environmental well-being.

---

3. Transforming Sustainable Practices Into Lifelong Habits

The journey of sustainable living is not a sprint but a marathon, and true change comes from building sustainable habits that last a lifetime. Transforming eco-friendly actions into habits requires patience, consistency, and the willingness to adapt, but the rewards are profound, both for personal well-being and the planetâ€™s health.

Tips for Sustaining Eco-Friendly Habits

- **Start with Small, Actionable Steps**: Begin by focusing on one habit at a time, such as composting food scraps or switching to eco-friendly cleaning products, and gradually build on each success.
- **Set Goals and Track Progress**: Set clear, achievable goals and track your progress to stay motivated and see how your actions contribute to a larger impact.
- **Create a Supportive Environment**: Surround yourself with reminders of your sustainable intentions, such as keeping reusable bags near the door or setting up a compost bin in the kitchen.
- **Celebrate Milestones**: Recognize and celebrate milestones, such as reducing household waste, lowering energy use, or completing a month of zero-waste practices. Celebrations reinforce commitment and keep the journey positive.

By turning sustainable actions into habits, we lay the foundation for a lifestyle that aligns with our values, creating a rhythm of mindfulness, care, and intentionality that extends into every aspect of life.

---

4. Embracing The Journey Of Lifelong Learning And Adaptation

Sustainable living is a dynamic field, constantly evolving as we discover new eco-friendly technologies, learn more about environmental issues, and adapt to the world's changing needs. Embracing this journey with a willingness to learn and grow allows us to make more informed, impactful choices over time. Each step we take builds on the last, creating a cycle of continuous improvement.

Strategies for Lifelong Learning in Sustainability

- **Stay Informed**: Follow environmental news, read books on sustainability, and engage with organizations that provide updates on eco-friendly innovations and climate science.
- **Adapt with Curiosity**: Embrace a mindset of curiosity, viewing new challenges as opportunities to learn and evolve your sustainable practices.
- **Participate in Workshops and Events**: Attend local workshops, online webinars, and community events focused on sustainability to connect with experts, gain practical skills, and stay motivated.
- **Share Knowledge and Experiences**: Engage in discussions with friends, family, and community members to share what you've learned and inspire others on their sustainability journey.

By committing to lifelong learning, we continue to adapt and grow, ensuring that our sustainable lifestyle remains relevant, effective, and fulfilling.

5. Cultivating Hope And Resilience For The Future

Hope and resilience are essential for sustaining a positive impact over the long term. Sustainable living requires perseverance in the face of environmental challenges, from climate change to pollution. By cultivating resilience, we empower ourselves to stay committed, overcome obstacles, and remain hopeful for the future we are building.

Practices to Cultivate Hope and Resilience

- **Celebrate Success Stories**: Read about successful conservation efforts, environmental victories, and community-led projects that have made a positive impact, reminding yourself that change is possible.
- **Focus on Solutions**: Instead of becoming overwhelmed by environmental issues, focus on solutions and actions you can take, from reducing waste to advocating for green policies.
- **Build a Resilient Mindset**: Embrace challenges as opportunities for growth and adaptability, developing a mindset that sees setbacks as part of the journey rather than the end.
- **Stay Connected to Nature**: Spend regular time outdoors, observing the beauty, resilience, and interconnectedness of natural ecosystems. Nature itself is a source of hope, inspiring us to protect and cherish it.

Cultivating hope and resilience sustains our energy, helping us remain dedicated to creating a world that values environmental health and harmony.

6. A Collective Vision: Building A Sustainable World Together

Our individual efforts are powerful, but our collective impact is transformative. When people come together with shared values and goals, the potential for positive change expands exponentially. By contributing to a collective vision of sustainability, we strengthen our communities, create lasting relationships, and support a culture that values the planet and its inhabitants.

Ways to Contribute to a Collective Vision

- **Engage in Community Projects**: Join or start community projects focused on sustainable initiatives, like community gardens, tree-planting events, or recycling drives. These projects amplify individual efforts, creating a shared vision for a sustainable neighborhood.
- **Advocate for Environmental Justice**: Support policies and initiatives that prioritize environmental equity, ensuring that all communities have access to clean air, water, and resources, regardless of socioeconomic background.
- **Educate and Inspire**: Share your knowledge and experiences with others, encouraging friends, family, and colleagues to embrace sustainable practices. Together, we can inspire a broader movement.
- **Support Sustainable Businesses and Organizations**: Choose to buy from companies and organizations committed to ethical practices, environmental health, and social responsibility, fostering a demand for sustainability on a larger scale.

By working together, we create a world where sustainable

living is not just a personal choice but a community value, strengthening our collective impact and fostering hope for future generations.

---

7. Final Reflections: A Vision for a Sustainable Future

As we conclude this book, remember that sustainable living is not an isolated journeyâ€"itâ€™s a way of life that connects us to each other, the Earth, and the generations to come. Each small action, each eco-friendly choice, and each shared experience contributes to a larger movement for a healthier, more resilient planet. Let this vision inspire you to continue your sustainable journey, knowing that your efforts are part of a global community working toward a brighter, greener future.

Guiding Principles for the Path Ahead

- **Embrace the Process**: Sustainable living is an ongoing process, filled with growth, reflection, and adaptation. Allow yourself to learn, evolve, and enjoy each step of the journey.
- **Seek Balance**: Sustainability is about balanceâ€"between self-care and environmental care, between personal goals and collective impact. Find a rhythm that nurtures both your well-being and your commitment to the Earth.
- **Honor Every Choice**: Every eco-friendly action, no matter how small, contributes to positive change. Honor each choice, recognizing it as a meaningful part of your journey.

These guiding principles remind us that sustainable living is a life of purpose, connection, and joy, offering fulfillment while making a positive impact.

Conclusion: Together Toward a Greener Tomorrow

As you close this book, know that you are equipped with the knowledge, tools, and inspiration to make a meaningful impact. Sustainable living is not just about the actions we take; it's about the legacy we create, the communities we strengthen, and the world we envision for the future.

Let each day be a celebration of progress, of purpose, and of the enduring beauty of the natural world. Embrace this journey with confidence and hope, knowing that each of us has the power to contribute to a brighter, more resilient tomorrow. Together, let's build a world where sustainable living is not just a choice but a way of life—a world that honors the Earth, nurtures our communities, and leaves a lasting legacy for generations to come.